Priority Setting and The Public

Penelope Mullen

and

Peter Spurgeon

Health Services Management Centre

University of Birmingham

Radcliffe Medical Press

© 2000 Penelope Mullen and Peter Spurgeon

Radcliffe Medical Press Ltd
18 Marcham Road, Abingdon, Oxon OX14 1AA

British Library Cataloguing in Publication Data

A catalogue record for this book is available from the British Library.

ISBN 1 85775 297 X

Typeset by Action Publishing Technology Ltd, Gloucester
Printed and bound by T J International Ltd, Padstow, Cornwall

Contents

Preface

In many societies the provision of appropriate healthcare according to need is viewed as morally correct – indeed a right – and the mark of a developed country, as well as being viewed as economically sound in helping to ensure a fit and productive workforce. Individual citizens place great value on such access. Thus talk of rationing – denying access to potentially beneficial healthcare – in the face of real or perceived imbalances of supply and demand, creates considerable concern. Nevertheless, various pressures (discussed in the text in Chapter One) have led to more and more explicit discussions of the need for some kind of priority-setting process to be established and to numerous attempts to set priorities. In viewing the debate, however, we became concerned at the apparently unquestioning acceptance of the need for 'hard choices', which overshadows the many aspects of healthcare provision and delivery where priority setting is both indicated and non-controversial. At the same time, from a rather more methodological point of view, we were concerned that many of the attempts at priority setting appeared to ignore longstanding experience within the healthcare sector and outside.

This book explores the reasons for the current pressure to set priorities and questions to a degree the assumed certainty of the arguments. It also explores and critically questions the role of public involvement in healthcare priority setting. It examines techniques and approaches used in priority setting, drawing on work both inside and outside the health sector. A review of the literature on priority setting is provided and this is then set in the context of practice, i.e. how the health service has set about the task of setting priorities and, particularly, how it has sought to involve the public in these processes. Considerable attention is given to the role of the public in priority setting as an ethical, conceptual and practical issue.

As international interest in priority setting continues to increase we hope that this book will provide a helpful guide to approaches in this area. It also asks some fundamental questions about what priority setting can achieve and suggests that we have to be very clear about the purpose and context in which we undertake priority setting.

We would like to acknowledge the financial support of The Nuffield Trust for the survey of priority-setting exercises reported in this book. Our thanks are also due to all the health service staff who participated in that survey and to colleagues at HSMC who have commented helpfully on earlier drafts. We are indebted to Sabrina Begum for her support in preparing and collating the material.

Finally, we hope the work will contribute to understanding and realism about priority setting and the role of the public in this process.

Penelope Mullen
Peter Spurgeon
September 1999

About the authors

Penelope Mullen is a Senior Lecturer at the Health Services Management Centre (HSMC), University of Birmingham, where she has responsibility for graduate programmes. Her background is in Operational Research and she worked as a Principal OR Officer in the NHS before joining the HSMC. She has researched and published widely in the areas of healthcare planning, resource allocation, performance indicators and waiting lists and, more recently, rationing and priority setting.

Peter Spurgeon is a psychologist by background and has worked in a number of sectors: universities, the computer industry and, most recently, health. He has particular interests in management and organisational development. His range of experience has been of particular value in supporting the extended management role of clinicians in the NHS.

He has published widely including texts on managing change and is the editor of the best-selling book *The New Face of The NHS*. For the past 10 years he has been the editor of the international journal *Health Services Management Research*.

Previously the Director of the HSMC, he is currently Director of Research.

CHAPTER ONE

The context of change in health systems

Introduction

Within the UK National Health Service (NHS) in recent years, in common with many other countries, there has been an upsurge of interest in explicit priority setting and also in the involvement of the public in decisions about healthcare provision. These two strands of thinking represent the focus of this text and will be explained in detail in subsequent chapters. However, priority setting is not merely a technical issue. It cannot be viewed in isolation from the rationing debate and priority setting within any healthcare system will be influenced, or even controlled, by the ideology of that system (Williams, 1988). Many of the forces providing an impetus to priority setting parallel the more general pressures to overall health system 'reform' or review. Therefore, before priority setting is examined specifically, a brief overview of the factors influencing health system 'reform' will be given.

The process of health system 'reform' is virtually universal in developed, and increasingly in developing, societies and by and large the forces advanced as promoting the 'reform' process are described in similar terms. They may be summarised as:

- a perceived need for governments to constrain the increasing costs of healthcare systems against a background of apparently ever-increasing demand
- rapid advances in medical technology and drugs which at once may increase short-term costs and radically change the way in which services are provided
- an increasing elderly population presenting complex multiple pathologies and requiring extended long-term care (Spurgeon, 1993).

In the UK, the previous Conservative government (through the 1980s and much of the 1990s) was driven in its attitude to public services by three fundamental and pervasive values or principles, which have particular importance for the subsequent interest in priority setting.

The first of these was a strong desire to move as much public sector provision as possible into the private sector, which was perceived by the government to be both more efficient and more responsive (Pollitt, 1986). Where that was not possible, there were attempts to introduce the 'disciplines' of the private sector and the market to the public sector.

This leads to the second principle, which was a strongly voiced concern for increased accountability at both institutional and personal levels, whereby public organisations were to be made more directly accountable for how public money was used. Clearly such financial scrutiny readily translates into questions of which health services should be purchased, whether this represents the best use of public money or whether alternative choices might have been made.

The third principle was the government's expressed desire to increase consumer choice, whether directly in respect of services received or by agents on behalf of the consumer. Once again, this desire has been translated into advocating an enhanced role for consumers (the public) in determining the nature of health services to be made available.

Such values were expressed through the creation of the 'internal market' in healthcare and were operationalised as:

- the separation of purchaser and provider roles with contracts or service agreements as the basis of the purchaser–provider relationship
- the establishment of NHS trusts as quasiautonomous organisations responsible for the provision of healthcare
- the creation of GP fundholding (GPFH), enabling some GPs to purchase a range of services on behalf of their registered patients.

It was hardly surprising that the 'reform' process contained inherent tension and conflict since the pre-1991 NHS had generally provided a comprehensive service with reasonable equity of access, with health outcomes comparable to other health systems, and at a total cost in 1990 of 6% of Total Domestic Expenditure (TDE) in the UK as compared to a European average of 7.5% of TDE (OECD, 1993). The 'reform' process should perhaps have been more appropriately targeted at those aspects of the NHS which might be described as rigid and unresponsive to pressures for change and lacking incentives for improvement in efficiency. A rather more extreme strategy to introduce a substantial element of private funding to supplement public expenditure (Letwin and Redwood, 1988) was rejected. Thus, in essence, the changes to the NHS were designed to change the delivery system to encourage greater efficiency, whilst preserving the basic method of financing the service and operating within the same broad financial parameters.

A very strong directional force to the subsequent priority-setting debate can be detected here with the explicit goal of obtaining greater value from a constrained budget. The expression of this choice mechanism through contracts set between purchasers and providers was in effect an attempt to obtain greater allocative efficiency (Posnett, 1993). Within the new NHS structure, both health authorities (HAs) and GP fundholders performed the purchasing function. The common feature of assessing the needs of their (resident or registered) population and then purchasing to meet those needs is the critical component relevant to priority setting. Both HAs and fundholders were charged with obtaining value for money and hence making choices between different types of healthcare provision. In a parallel process, providers were to organise themselves to respond to purchaser requirements and to compete against one another to secure contracts by providing services in the most efficient and cost-effective manner.

The expressed intention of the separation of the purchasing function from the provision of healthcare was to provide greater freedom and independence for the purchaser in planning contracts in the best interests of the population rather than the vested interests of the provider organisation. The fact that this did not really happen other than at the periphery was largely due to the immaturity of purchasing as a function within the NHS and also to the major imperfections of healthcare as a market environment (Spurgeon, 1997).

Nonetheless, it is fair to say that within an overall budget framework, purchasers began to set priorities for treatment, to evaluate the cost-effectiveness of alternative procedures and to develop measures of healthcare outcomes as part of the process of monitoring and evaluating the performance of suppliers. The documentation of contracts was increasingly making priority setting more transparent and open to public scrutiny – and concern (Moore, 1996). Recent high-profile cases relating to the cost of new drugs such as interferon-β for multiple sclerosis sufferers (Zimmern, 1995) and the denial of treatment to Child B by her health authority (New and Le Grand, 1996) are examples of both the process of priority setting at work and the potential volatility of public reaction once such decisions become explicit.

Continuing processes of 'reform' and factors increasing the interest in priority setting

Ever since the inception of the NHS, access to healthcare has been restricted in one form or another. These restrictions, which are now frequently termed 'implicit rationing', have taken a variety of forms including waiting and raising the threshold for treatment. However, the inception of the 'internal market' was accompanied by an increasing interest in 'explicit rationing', which is usually understood to mean deciding explicitly which services or treatments will be provided by the NHS and which will not (for examples, see Brindle, 1995a, c; RCP, 1995). Whilst this had always been done to some extent at the national level, by declaring that certain forms of treatment or drugs were not available on the NHS, the new focus on rationing was found at the level of the purchaser (HA or GP fundholder).

The major reason for this change in decision-making focus lay in alterations to the way hospitals and other healthcare providers were funded. Under the old pre-1991

NHS, hospitals were directly funded and managed by their HAs. Planners and politicians could influence priorities by determining which facilities/services to provide and their location, thus restricting access both by capacity and by distance. But within the overall resource allocation, most 'rationing' was controlled by clinicians, via waiting and thresholds. Under the post-1991 contract-based system, with the purchaser–provider split described above, purchasers were able to determine explicitly, and in some detail, what services/treatments they would and would not purchase for their resident or registered populations. This opened up the possibility of explicit rationing which some, for instance Ham (1998), argue is a better system than the implicit rationing of the past.

However, it must also be acknowledged that such an approach may also act as a shield to politicians unwilling to be seen to restrict services themselves and preferring to place other organisations in the battleground of withdrawal of health provision. Moreover, with greater explicitness, a rigidity in decision making is introduced, necessitating guidelines, protocols, criteria, etc., unlike previous approaches which, although somewhat fuzzy, may have had greater scope to absorb difficult decisions. This is an issue we will return to in later chapters.

The problems and opportunities afforded by the purchaser–provider split are likely to continue. The Labour government, which was elected in May 1997, stated in the White Paper *The New NHS* (DoH, 1997) its intention to abolish the *internal market* introduced by the previous government. However, decisions on which services to 'purchase' or 'commission' will remain at local level, mainly in the hands of primary care groups (PCGs), led by general practitioners and responsible for populations of around 100 000, with HAs performing a co-ordinating and strategic planning function.

Certainly, the move from 'implicit' to 'explicit' rationing has created a vast range of debates and controversy. The separation of purchaser from provider, although a major contributor in the factors leading to increased interest in priority setting, is not the sole impetus. A number of other developments in healthcare systems have served to reinforce this process.

National priorities and planning guidelines

The Priorities and Planning Guidance 1997–98 issued to the service by the NHS Executive in 1996 (NHSE, 1996a) attempted to provide an overall context for the planning and delivery of health services and to focus local decision makers on the most important national priorities. The content of the guidelines is not really the point and, indeed, they have been changed by the incoming Labour administration. Their importance is to be seen in the relationship between national government and the local allocators of resources. The latter, HAs and purchasing GPs, are aware that they will be monitored in terms of their performance against national priorities. Thus, where such priorities require additional resources in order to be achieved, it is immediately possible that decisions may be needed to redirect resources to these target areas, i.e. priorities will have to be set.

In addition, nationally determined Patient's Charter standards, such as waiting-time targets, can create prioritisation decisions – or distortions, as some would argue. Finally, national guidelines are frequently supplemented by within-year imperatives, so clearly purchasing strategies must operationalise some form of priority setting in order to balance delivery against these (often competing) goals.

Healthcare needs assessment

Purchasers have a responsibility to meet the needs of their population, whether resident or registered, but the concept of need is subjective, dynamic and multi-dimensional. There is a major area of debate and discussion surrounding the concept of need and it cannot be covered in depth here. However, the debate around needs assessment neatly exemplifies some of the competing perspectives which must be reconciled if an acceptable priority-setting process is to emerge.

Possibly the dominant perspective is that based on the epidemiological/medical approach, which equates health need with the presence of disease in a population (Foreman, 1996). Thus the extent of illness is used as a basis to assess both need for health and need for healthcare. However, Culyer and Wagstaff (1993, p.434), who examine a number of definitions of need, are especially critical of the argument that 'persons who are more ill than others have a greater need', a notion that underlies many of the empirical studies. They suggest that 'it is hard to see why someone who is sick can sensibly be said to need health care, irrespective of the latter's ability to improve the person's health'.

The notion of 'capacity to benefit' leads to the second perspective, widely advocated by health economists, which places much greater emphasis upon the cost-effective-ness of treatments. This leads to the argument that resources should be allocated and priorities set in order to maximise the total benefit obtained from those resources; resources should be allocated to those treatments and services which achieve the most quality-adjusted life years (QALYs) per pound.

The rather technical aspect of that approach is in contrast to the third perspective (the social approach) which is more holistic and seeks to incorporate aspects of an indi-vidual's social, economic and environmental situation. This perspective is associated with definitions of health which go beyond the 'absence of disease', as exemplified by the World Health Organisation definition: 'a state of complete physical, mental and social well-being and not merely the absence of disease or infirmity'. Daniels (1985, p.32) suggests that 'Health care needs will be those things we need in order to main-tain, restore, or provide functional equivalents (where possible) to normal species functioning', impairments to which, he argues (p.27), 'reduce the range of opportu-nity open to the individual'. This range – the normal opportunity range – 'for a given society is the array of life plans reasonable persons in it are likely to construct for themselves' (p.33) and is thus dependent on key features of that society including historical and technological development, material wealth and culture.

Foreman (1996, p.69) argues that 'While the epidemiological and social models would attempt to meet all the needs that fall within their respective definitions, the economic model effectively replaces needs with the more restricted concept of priorities'. The latter model has gained some ascendancy in recent years. In many senses, the arguments surrounding the health-maximising approach capture the essence of the priority-setting tension: how far should healthcare systems seek to meet needs as defined by the social and/or medical approaches as opposed to focusing on the most cost-effective interventions?

Primary care-led services

Along with many countries, the UK has seen a proliferation of initiatives designed to shift the focus from secondary to primary care. Despite assumptions by some proponents of a primary care-led NHS that healthcare provision by generalists rather than specialists and an enhanced gatekeeper role for primary care will be cheaper, it is as yet unproven that such a shift will result in reduced costs (Audit Commission, 1996; Coote and Hunter, 1996). Indeed, a better resourced primary care sector may actually increase demand on specialist secondary care. Whilst evidence accumulates and debate continues around the issue, it is clear that in order to support the expansion of primary care within a constrained budget, decisions about the size and activity of the secondary sector will need to be taken. This leads again to the issue of priority setting.

Evidence-based medicine

Both the previous and current governments in the UK have placed great emphasis upon delivering a knowledge-based health service. There are two key reasons given for this.

• If the rationing of scarce resources requires resources to be targeted at the most effective interventions, it is necessary to have appropriate evidence as to which these are.

• The large variations observed in clinical practice are assumed to represent a wasteful use of resources, which might otherwise be used to provide alternative and better services (Grimshaw and Hutchinson, 1995).

A belief underlying the move to evidence-based medicine is that if rigorous scientific evaluation is applied to current and new treatments, ineffective treatments can be discontinued, costs can be reduced and effectiveness increased. It has been suggested that up to £1 billion of resources could be released by withdrawing from unnecessary and ineffective treatments (New and Le Grand, 1996).

The view that savings will inevitably arise is not universal, with Sackett (1996) suggesting that costs may actually increase as a result of evidence-based medicine and Appleby (1995) pointing out that the process of assessing the evidence has focused mainly on whether interventions work rather than their cost-effectiveness. In many clinical contexts the existing evidence is equivocal and many clinicians will argue that guidelines and information stimulate as many questions as they resolve. Nonetheless, the knowledge-based practice concept provides further impetus to the need to understand the priority-setting process.

Indeed, the whole argument around the effectiveness of clinical interventions has been intense and emotive. What appear to be rational decisions about the reconfiguration of services to develop centres of excellence with a critical mass of expertise have encountered strong opposition to the loss of access to local provision. Thus, even where services are maintained, in total, the location of services has become a further issue of contention for purchasers in defining the pattern and nature of services at specific sites.

Priorities in practice

Finally, an empirical study of priority setting in practice (Im, 1998) revealed that the most important considerations for HAs in establishing their purchasing priorities were:

- assessing local needs
- evidence of cost-effectiveness
- listening to the views of local GPs
- improving efficiency/value for money.

Maintaining existing patterns of services was viewed as the least important aspect. This contrast between what is seen as important and what is not provides real evidence of the dynamic for change. Least influential is maintaining the status quo whilst all the factors we have described above emerge as key forces for altering services and for setting priorities.

It is clear from this brief overview that 'reform' processes and initiatives in the health system have served to focus attention on the need for priority setting. Indeed, it could be argued that choices, if not rationing, are inevitable in the process of providing health services. It is also clear that such choices occur at different levels within health systems and that again, almost inevitably, such decisions will involve conflicts with each other. This is especially likely when population needs are compared to the best interests of the individual patient. It is also clear that organisations are approaching priority setting in a variety of ways and that expertise in techniques is very variable.

These issues will be explained in more depth throughout this text. Chapter Two examines the concepts relating to the rationing process and academic contributions to this debate. Chapters Three, Four and Five trace the practice of consumer involvement in the health system through to priority setting and how health organisations might engage with the public in this task. Chapter Six identifies a range of possible methods which could be used and these are given practical expression in Chapter Seven, which reports the findings from a survey of what health organisations are doing and examples of what has been achieved. Finally, in Chapter Eight, the future of healthcare is considered in the context of priority-setting issues.

CHAPTER TWO

Setting priorities and healthcare rationing

Priority setting and rationing

Over recent years, priority setting in healthcare has been overshadowed by the more emotive term 'rationing'. In a world where not all activities can be carried out simultaneously, some form of sequencing or prioritisation is inevitable. However, despite the claim by Salter (1993, p.173) that 'Priority setting is after all rationing by any other name in that it is a statement about the selective allocation of scarce resources in a situation of excess demand over supply', not all priority setting in healthcare is associated with or necessarily leads to the denial currently associated with the term 'rationing'.

Klein *et al.* (1995, p.770) suggest that, in principle if not always in practice, 'rationing is to be distinguished from priority setting'. 'While the former affects individual patients, the latter involves allocating resources to specific services or client groups', adding that priority setting provides the parameters within which rationing takes place. It is not clear how useful this distinction is and, in any case, it suggests too narrow a definition of priority setting which can range from the relatively neutral prioritisation of the sequence of linear activities, mentioned above, to the more emotive elimination or denial of healthcare considered low priority, which is frequently associated with rationing.

Nevertheless, the healthcare rationing debate is now so widespread in the UK, and has spawned such an enormous literature, that it is impossible to discuss priority setting and priority-setting approaches without at least noting the overshadowing rationing debate.

What is healthcare rationing?

Despite the widespread debate on healthcare rationing, many UK commentators simply use the word 'rationing' – undefined – and proceed with the discussion from there. There is often little attempt to define what is meant by rationing but, nevertheless, it quickly becomes apparent that different commentators are interpreting it in different ways.

However, despite the suggestion above that the term 'rationing' is now considered emotive, rationing still carries for many the wartime notion of fairness, where food rationing was instituted to ensure equitable allocation of a scarce commodity, rather than allowing allocation by market price. This notion is picked up by some commentators in the US literature, where there seems a far greater propensity to seek definitions of rationing. For instance, Fleck (1992) turns to Reagan's (1990, p.223) definition of rationing as 'a mode of non-price distribution of particular services among particular individuals' which 'is "inherently" comparative . . . [as] . . . community policy makers seek to achieve equitable distribution of what is a scarce resource'. Mechanic (1985, p.457) states that 'Rationing is no more than a means of apportioning, through some method of allowance, some limited good or service'.

However, turning specifically to healthcare, a more emotive tone is detected in the US literature. Relman (1990, p.1809) defines the ideas of rationing now being proposed as 'the deliberate and systematic denial of certain types of services, even when they are known to be beneficial', which he contrasts with the kind of rationing by 'global government budgetary restraints on facilities and personnel, such as occurs in centrally planned health economies like those of Great Britain or Sweden'.

Nelson and Drought (1992, p.101) offer 'withholding necessary interventions from patients', whilst Dougherty (1991, p.3) states that health services prioritisation implies 'a form of health care rationing, that is, the denial of services that are potentially beneficial to some people because of limitations on the resources available for health care. This means putting the common good ahead of the interests of individuals in some cases'.

Fleck (1992, p.1605) claims that 'rationing means that government will deny one of its citizens life-sustaining medical care on the basis of an arbitrary budgetary limit', whilst Hadorn and Brook (1991, p.3331) define rationing as 'the societal toleration of inequitable access to health services acknowledged to be necessary by reference to necessary-care guidelines'.

Similar definitions are appearing in the UK literature, with Klein *et al.* (1995, p.770) stating that 'rationing involves the denial or dilution of something that is potentially beneficial to the patient: he or she is getting less in the way of treatment than might be thought desirable in a world with unlimited resources'.

Although many of these definitions may appear somewhat emotive, what they do make clear is that 'the elimination of care that provides no benefits at all' (Aaron, 1992, p.107) does not constitute rationing.

Most discussion about healthcare rationing is, implicitly or explicitly, concerned only with the rationing of publicly funded healthcare. However, some US commentators see rationing more widely as denying access to services for which the potential beneficiaries are willing and able to pay. Pawlson *et al.* (1992, p.629) draw on the analogy of wartime petrol rationing and suggest that 'Rationing is also sometimes used in a very restricted sense to refer only to situations in which specific individuals or groups are denied access to services that are of benefit and for which they could pay'. Following the same line, Aaron (1992, p.107) states:

> *I use it [the word rationing] to mean the denial to people who have the means to pay for healthcare [of] some services that promise medical benefits. By that definition, the denial of care to those who are uninsured is not what I call rationing.*

The argument is taken further by distinguishing between the rationing of healthcare and the rationing of healthcare finance:

> *rules restricting the availability of health care financing ... however, ration only health care financing, not medical care itself. Thus a service that is deemed to fall outside a patient's coverage is not necessarily denied to the patient. It may still be provided at the patient's personal expense or at the expense of the provider ... (Havighurst, 1992, p.1759)*

By contrast, Brown (1991, p.30) states that rationing means 'the deliberate, systematic withholding of beneficial goods or services from some elements of the population on the grounds that society cannot afford to extend them'.

Drawing on the classification of different forms of rationing represented by the five Ds – Deterrence, Delay, Deflection, Dilution, Denial – originating from Parker (1967), we see that the definitions above focus largely on Denial, which may account for some of the emotion now surrounding the notion of rationing. This is also closely associated with the debate surrounding *explicit* rationing versus *implicit* rationing. *Explicit* rationing, which is often associated with open and explicit statements about which treatments will and will not be supplied or which patients will or will not be treated, is advocated by many as superior to *implicit* rationing, which is usually associated with waiting for treatment, limiting numbers of tests and raising thresholds for treatment within global budgets.

Is healthcare rationing necessary?

Many commentators consider the need for rationing to be axiomatic (Rivlin, 1997, p.113 *inter alia*), and thus that the only issue is how that rationing should be carried out. The Rationing Agenda Group (New, 1996, p.1594), although claiming 'to present the issues, not take up positions on them', base their presentation on the 'substantive view' that rationing is inevitable. Indeed, in the US context, Califano (1992, p.1525) suggests that 'a growing number of politicians and health care experts seem bent on elevating health care rationing to a national policy'.

Some commentators, however, question the whole notion of rationing healthcare at all. They claim that healthcare rationing is unnecessary and a diversion from the real problem of the funding and delivery of healthcare. Further, they argue that the automatic acceptance of the need for rationing leads to pessimism and a series of undesirable consequences. In Califano's (1992, p.1538) view, 'Rationing is not a solution to the problems we face, it is a capitulation of despair'. These arguments are anathema to those who see rationing as axiomatic, those who claim resources will always be scarce and rationing is inevitable. Challengers of the necessity for rationing are accused of not living in the real world.

However, Light (1997, p.113) suggests that:

> to say 'that rationing is inevitable and therefore we should focus on how to ration reasonably' is like the medical professional deciding that 'death is inevitable and therefore we should focus on how to die reasonably'. Death is inevitable, but the conclusion denies the whole purpose of medicine.

An element of machismo enters the language at this point with talk of tough decisions and hard choices. For instance, Arcangelo (1994, p.25) states: 'Tough decisions must be made about allocation of services', whilst Brown (1991, p.31) suggests business executives see rationing as meaning tackling 'hard choices' – which they suppose to be good. The UK debate on rationing is also peppered with references to the necessity of facing hard choices. For instance, the preamble to an article on HA priority setting by Redmayne (1992, p.28), which itself repeatedly mentions 'hard choices', contains the somewhat value-laden statement that 'health authorities are avoiding difficult decisions about rationing by tinkering at the edges'. 'Hard choices' has appeared in the title of conferences and books (Lenaghan, 1997). It is almost as if a new value system has arisen which equates explicit rationing with hard and thus strong, good decision making, while implicit rationing is characterised as soft and thereby associated with weak, poor decision making. Those who deny the need to ration and those who advocate implicit rationing within global budgets are accused of weakness and simply trying to avoid these hard choices.

Similar dichotomised thinking was evident in the early stages of the separation of the purchasing of healthcare from its provision in the UK. Many purchasers interpreted their role in rather macho terms, seeing their task as 'sorting out' inefficient providers. This somewhat immature approach has gradually retreated and a more mature approach may infiltrate future rationing debates.

There does, however, appear to be a move to rehabilitate the concept of rationing. Lenaghan (1996a, p.8) regrets that 'far too many people use the term rationing as if it were a negative process', preferring to see it as a positive process to ensure fair distribution of finite resources. Heginbotham (1997, p.45) notes that some people find the term 'rationing' uncomfortable, seeing it to be synonymous with cuts, reductions, insufficient care and 'with the idea that unpalatable and tough decisions have to be taken'. He suggests that although 'rationing is linked to the need for tough decisions', it is also an ethical word.

The question of whether rationing is necessary appears to become less clearcut the more closely it is considered. Despite a little cynicism about the motives of some participants, it is interesting to note the change in voting at a debate in March 1993, organised by the BMA. Held under Cambridge Union Rules, the debate was on the motion 'This house believes that rationing in healthcare is inevitable'. Before the debate, the voting was: For 110, Against 22, Abstentions 7. After the debate it was: For 68, Against 65, Abstentions 3.

Challenges to assumption of the 'inevitability of healthcare rationing' include arguments that rationing would not be necessary if there were greater efficiency, if non-effective treatment were eliminated or if the NHS were properly funded. Possibly more fundamental, however, is the challenge to the assertion that healthcare demand, or need, is infinite and that resources are finite, which is the most common argument for the inevitability or necessity of rationing. Indeed, Julian Tudor Hart coined the phrase 'finite need – infinite resources' which, whilst not intended to be pushed to extremes, challenges and turns round the oft-quoted phrase 'infinite needs – finite resources' and serves to prompt questioning of the original formulation.

Is demand/need infinite?

Many who claim rationing as inevitable do so on the grounds that demand, or even need, for healthcare is infinite (see, for instance, Salter, 1994, p.48). Roberts *et al.* (1995a) observe that the:

> statement that 'the demand for healthcare is infinite, and therefore rationing is inevitable', is now used so often that the public may come to believe it uncritically, and so accept any consequent policy recommendations.

Efforts at rationing are 'commonly informed by the pessimistic belief that the satisfaction of demand is an unrealistic goal' (Frankel, 1991, p. 1590).

The notion of infinite need, if not infinite demand, can be challenged by the observation that both the amount of disease and the number of people who are, or could be, suffering from that disease are finite. Williams and Frankel (1993, p.15), questioning the existence of the unmet iceberg of need, ask 'can any reasonable level of health care provision satisfy the needs of the population?' and, in the case of particular healthcare requirements at least, answer in the affirmative. They support their argument by reference to studies from the Epidemiological Based Needs Assessment Research Programme, which suggest a finite, measurable and deliverable level of need for particular treatments. Roberts *et al.* (1995a) claim that the 'need' for effective healthcare is finite and that a range of factors are contributing to the idea that need (or demand) for healthcare is infinite. After detailed discussion of various aspects of healthcare, Rawles (1989, p.144) concludes that demand is not infinite and 'in many cases ... could be completely satisfied with just a modest increase in resources'.

Infinite or at least excessive demand, as Aaron and Schwartz (1990, p.418) point out, is seen by many as an inevitable consequence of a third-party payer, with healthcare being free to the patient at point of delivery. However, a zero monetary price at the point of service delivery does not mean that the recipient incurs no cost (in terms of time, inconvenience, lost earnings, etc.) in securing that service. But even if services are totally costless to recipients, there is no theoretical or practical support for arguments that they would (wish to) consume infinite amounts of that service. Economists would argue that demand would cease when the marginal utility fell to zero. Commonsense would suggest that we do not all wish to consume healthcare simply because it is there. However, Healthcare 2000 (1995, p.40) states simply that 'we believe that it is inevitable that rationing will take place for those services provided free or at low price to users'.

The expanding range of new healthcare technologies has been cited as a cause of escalating health service costs. However, although there is general agreement that the growth in technological developments in healthcare will continue, it is also argued that some new developments (e.g. minimally invasive surgery, drug therapies replacing surgery) might prove more cost-effective than existing treatments (Hunter, 1992). After reviewing various empirical results, Wordsworth *et al.* (1996, p.18) conclude that 'although the future of the NHS partially depends on new technology, not all of that technology will be cost increasing'. However, Harrison *et al.* (1997, p.140), suggesting that lack of relevant research means that it 'is hard to find examples where new technologies have reduced spending in the health system as a whole rather than on individual patients', point out that 'the introduction and use of technology is to some extent amenable to control'. Nevertheless, even if new technologies do not lead to the escalating costs feared by some, they may prove, on balance, to be cost increasing. Rawles (1989, p.144), however, suggests that even if the figure of 2% above inflation, commonly estimated as being needed to keep up with increases in demand from technological change, increasing numbers of elderly and policy changes, is wrong, it is a long way short of infinity.

Demographic trends, which indicate an ageing of the population, are widely cited as another reason for predicting an escalation in demand for healthcare. Yet, according to Defever (1991, p.1), 'a variety of persistent myths, nurtured by an amazing blindness for facts' characterise healthcare for the elderly and lead to conclusions about unbearable costs.

On the basis that per capita healthcare spending is far higher for older age groups, especially the over-85s, than for younger adults, it is commonly assumed that the increasing numbers in these older age groups will result in a dramatic increase in healthcare costs. However, even on its own terms, this prediction is disputed by Harrison *et al.* (1997, p.139). They applied constant age-specific per capita spending rates to the population projections for 2040 and estimated that a real increase in NHS spending of 8.25% between 1994 and 2014 would be required to cope with demographic change. This, they note, is less than the estimated growth of 10.3% between 1974 and 1994. Further, however, it has been demonstrated that this methodology is likely to produce a considerable overestimate of the effects of ageing (Getzen, 1992, p. 99).

The effect of increasing numbers of very elderly people on healthcare expenditure has been widely overestimated for a variety of reasons. It is observed that a large proportion of morbidity, and thus healthcare expenditure, is concentrated in the last few months of life (Fries, 1984, 1989). This suggests that the higher per capita healthcare costs for the very elderly are, at least partly, explained by the cost of dying and thus it is incorrect to calculate the increase in healthcare costs pro rata to the increase in the number of elderly people in each age group. Indeed, in so far as the increased proportion of the elderly in the population is due to longevity rather than reductions in the birth rate, assumptions that age-specific healthcare costs from the past can be projected into the future are somewhat alarming. In doing this, the implicit assumption is that the additional years of life will be accompanied by the average morbidity patterns experienced at that age by earlier generations, i.e. the additional years of life will be additional years of ill health not additional healthy years. Evidence on this is disputed but a US study by Fries *et al.* (1992), comparing intergenerational health status between parents and children at the same age, showed marked and significant evidence of decreasing age-specific morbidity over time. Wilson (1991) suggests that the 'terminal drop' model of ageing – the retention of independence and relatively good health until the final, dramatic fall in health status leading to death – 'is now that reality for the majority of old people' (p.45).

The 'compression of morbidity' hypothesis (Fries, 1980):

> *envisions ... postponing the age of onset of chronic infirmity relative to average life duration so that the period of morbidity is compressed between an increasing age of onset and a relatively fixed life expectancy.* (Fries, 1989, p.208)

If this thesis is correct – and it is disputed (Schneider and Brody, 1983 *inter alia*) – it would further reduce the anticipated pressure on healthcare expenditure caused by an ageing population. However, analysis by Bone *et al.* (1995) suggests little evidence of the compression of morbidity in respect of lower levels of disability, suggesting that 'Future gains in life expectancy among elderly people may well be accompanied by a rise in the amount of chronic disability' (p.33). However, in respect of severe disability – inability to perform Activities of Daily Living (ADLs) independently – there is evidence of a compression of morbidity (p.30). Indeed, they present figures (p.29) which suggest that for each of the older age groups (over 75), the percentage unable to perform ADLs independently dropped dramatically between 1976 and 1991.

A further challenge to the assumption that an ageing population leads to increasing healthcare expenditure is found in analysis of healthcare expenditure in 20 countries (Getzen, 1992). Using cross-sectional and time-series analyses, once inflation and national income are taken into account, no association was found between either total healthcare expenditure or the rate of change in healthcare expenditure and the proportion of the population aged over 65. Graphs showing (a) healthcare share of GNP plotted against the percentage of the population age 65+ and (b) the increasing health expenditures as a share of GDP plotted against the increase in the percentage of the population age 65+ dramatically illustrate the lack of correlation between ageing and healthcare costs (Getzen, 1992, p.102).

However, another aspect of demographic change, the reducing pool of informal carers (Wordsworth *et al.*, 1996, p.6), may result in increased costs falling on the NHS.

To recognise that neither the need nor the demand for healthcare is infinite may help to dispel the fatalism that pervades many arguments; that since need/demand is infinite, we might as well give up trying to meet it and start making the 'hard choices' of rationing. However, even if it is accepted that need/demand is finite, there is still the problem of determining the size of that finite need/demand. Studies such as those carried out under the Epidemiological Needs Assessment Research Programme (mentioned above) are attempting to quantify the level of need for specific treatments.

Light (1997, p.113), attacking the claim of a bottomless pit of health needs as 'a myth and an indefensible form of paternalism', suggests that 'the depth of the pit can be determined by taking people in a well funded healthcare system who face no barriers of time, distance, money, or delays and measuring their rates of surgery, or drug use, or visits to the doctor'. He has suggested (Light, 1995) that urban, middle-class, retired Germans might constitute an appropriate group for such an exercise. He further points out (1997, p.113) that although the Dutch and Germans do have more operations and doctor visits than the British, 'the rates are far from infinite'.

To sum up in Frankel's (1991, p.1590) words:

The assumptions that underlie this pessimism [about the inability to satisfy demand] should be questioned, and abandoned in favour of empirical determination of health-care requirements, with the assumption that there may be no need to ration those interventions of undoubted efficacy.

Are resources finite?

The question of finite resources for healthcare is often posed in terms of publicly funded healthcare. This specific point will be addressed below. The wider question here must be: is it possible to provide sufficient healthcare to satisfy the needs of the population? That is, can (not, at this point, does it wish to) society afford to devote to healthcare sufficient of its (real) resources, whether funded publicly or privately, to meet this requirement?

Of course, some resources, such as organs for transplant, are by their nature *absolutely scarce* (Fleck, 1995b, p.877). The concern here is with resources that are *fiscally scarce*: those whose scarcity, according to Fleck, 'is a result of a social/institutional decision to make no more money available for the purchase of that good to save lives under those circumstances'.

A more fundamental question than what publicly funded healthcare a society can or wishes to afford is whether total (private and public) expenditure on healthcare is, or is likely to become, so high that it causes serious damage to the rest of the economy. This question is most frequently posed in respect of the US where, Hackler (1993, p.5) points out, without 'serious structural changes' total healthcare spending is predicted to rise to 17% of GDP by 2000 and 37% by 2030. Hackler continues that 'As more of our money goes to health care, less is available for other critical social needs, such as education and economic investment'. Etzioni (1991, p.88) suggests, however, that Fuchs' (1990, p.534) argument that the increase in healthcare expenditure 'has a particularly traumatic effect on other sectors' is far from self-evident. There is no reason to suggest that any particular percentage of GNP is the correct amount to spend on health.

Etzioni also points out that advocates of healthcare rationing, who support their argument by showing that health costs have risen faster than inflation, 'neglect to mention that this is typical of services compared to the price of commodities'. Aaron and Schwartz (1990, p.418) similarly point to the 'tendency for the price of services characterized by low growth in productivity to rise relative to the price of commodities'. Baumol (1995, p.17) uses a musical example to illustrate this point. 'It is the relatively stagnant technology of live musical performance – its inherent resistance to productivity improvements – that accounts for the compounding rise in the cost of performance of quartets.' In his elegant exposition, Baumol (1995) argues that if those working in labour-intensive 'handicraft' industries with little potential for productivity increases are not to see their relative standard of living fall, then the share of GDP devoted to services such as health and education must rise. This, he demonstrates, is not only consistent with, but an inevitable consequence of, an overall increase in productivity and prosperity within the national economy.

This line of argument suggests that concern about the share of GDP devoted to health (and indeed education) may be misplaced. If the relative labour inputs of different sectors of the economy change, it would be expected *mutatis mutandis* that the relative shares of GDP accounted for by those different sectors will also change. Indeed, the only way that the share of GDP devoted to labour-intensive sectors can be held constant in the face of productivity increases in the capital-intensive sectors is by reducing the labour input and/or reducing the relative price of that labour. The effect of differential changes in productivity or labour input, which appears not to be sufficiently considered in debates on healthcare expenditure, may indeed be a major contributory factor to the well-documented relationship between per capita GDP and the percentage of GDP devoted to health services.

Concern about the level of the total expenditure on health has led to some advocacy of rationing of privately funded healthcare. Wiener (1992, p.13) notes that 'What is new in the debate is that people are beginning to talk about rationing for the insured as well as for the uninsured' and Honigsbaum (1991, p.9) reports that the initiators of the Oregon plan want it 'to set a pattern not only for the poor but for the population in general', an aspect that appears to have been rather overshadowed in the subsequent debate on Oregon.

In the US context, the argument has been made that the total share of resources devoted to health is so excessive that it is objectively damaging the rest of the economy. This, however, is countered by Etzioni (1991, p.88), who states that 'arguments that the United States is spending "too much" on health care are based in part on value judgements and must be judged accordingly'. Wiener (1992, p.19) supports this by claiming that there is 'nothing magic about 11–13 percent of the gross national product that says the world will collapse if we spend more than that'. 'Indeed,' he continues, 'a strong argument can be made that money spent on health care is morally preferable to some alternative uses, such as expensive cars, designer clothes, and fancy jewelry.' Baumol (1993, p.21) claims that 'Contrary to appearances, we *can* afford ever more ample medical care, ever more abundant education ... along with a growing profusion of private comforts and luxuries. It is an *illusion* that we cannot do so ...'

Turning to the UK context, where total expenditure on healthcare – public and private – consumes a vastly lower share of GDP, there appears to be little argument that aggregate resource use by healthcare is so high as to damage the economy. Further, the implications of the differential potential for productivity increases between labour-intensive industries and capital-intensive industries, discussed above, appear to have received little attention. It is, however, fair to conclude that any limit on total healthcare expenditure in the UK is a matter of choice, not economic necessity. How much, in total, should be devoted to healthcare is not a given.

Although this discussion has focused on *fiscal scarcity*, as noted earlier, some resources such as organs for transplant and, in the short term, facilities such as intensive care units are *absolutely scarce* and thus rationing is unavoidable. But, are there other real resources which are also *absolutely scarce* in the sense that their use by the health sector in competition with other sectors of the economy would damage those sectors? The major resource used in health services is labour – a resource not currently in short supply in most developed countries. Further, skilled labour is largely created by education, another labour-intensive sector. It is thus unlikely that expanding health services in the UK and other developed countries would deprive other sectors of the economy of *absolutely scarce* resources.

Despite the concern of some, especially in the US, about the level of total resources devoted to healthcare, most discussion about 'finite' resources and rationing relates to publicly funded healthcare. Indeed, it is claimed that rationing is inevitable in all systems of publicly funded healthcare (Emson, 1991), whilst Harrison (1997, p.131) goes further and extends that inevitability to 'any system of third party payment for health care'.

The level of expenditure on a publicly funded healthcare system is, however, not a given. It is a value or political judgement, a societal choice. There is no absolute limit other than one which might apply to total expenditure on healthcare, as discussed above. As Hart (1994, p.22) puts it:

The level of state funding depends on real rather than rhetorical social priorities. If suffi-cient private wealth exists for the whole population to pay individually for medical

services in the market, it must exist also as a potential tax base for services to be paid for
collectively . . .

Turning specifically to the NHS, it has been argued that there would be no need to
ration healthcare in the UK if the NHS were funded at a level nearer to that of other
developed countries. Similar arguments are levelled in the US by critics of the Oregon
plan, who point out that Oregon ranks 46th out of 50 states in its level of expenditure
on Medicaid (Brannigan, 1993), whilst Aaron (1992) claims that it would be relatively inexpensive to provide care to uninsured Americans at the average level
available to the insured.

However, Klein (1993, p.309) notes that in the Netherlands, where 8% of GDP was
spent on healthcare in 1990, there is a debate about rationing healthcare. Thus, he
claims, it would be 'dangerous to assume that there would be no need for rationing if
only Britain spent a higher proportion of the national income on health care'.
However, to conclude from that that there would be no benefit from increasing the
NHS's share of GDP, as it would/might not 'eliminate rationing', is equivalent to
arguing that it would make no difference if the NHS's share of GDP were cut substantially.

As Rawles (1989, p.143) says of the NHS, 'it is not obvious why resources have to
be rigidly fixed at the present inadequate level'. MacKay (1996), in a letter to the *BMJ*,
claims that there 'is no shortage of money in Britain, but we have become the victims
of political rhetoric and are beginning to believe the politicians' assertions that we
cannot afford a national health service, that as tax payers we are not prepared to pay
for a comprehensive service, and that such a service would require endless amounts of
money'. Advocates of an adequate level of funding for the NHS have argued that 'It is
obscene to deny care in a society where most people can afford luxuries and fripperies
and where some people are exceedingly affluent' (ACHCEW, 1993, p.33).

Efficiency and the cost of provision

It is frequently argued that there would be no (or possibly less) need for rationing if
inefficiencies in the healthcare system were eliminated (Roberts *et al.*, 1995b). Whilst
this argument is posed most strongly in the context of the US health system (Etzioni,
1991), intraspecialty cost variations are cited as evidence of the potential for cost
saving and greater efficiency in the NHS (ACHCEW, 1993).

However, in the US context it is claimed that eliminating inefficiencies results only
in 'one-off' savings and would not halt the rise in healthcare costs (Aaron and
Schwartz, 1990). Further, Fleck (1994a) argues that most proposals to increase efficiency would, in fact, constitute implicit rationing. On the other hand, Califano (1992,
p.1526) argues that the US expenditure of $800 billion is more than enough to
provide all health and long-term care Americans need '. . . with a little efficiency,
prudence and prevention'.

High administrative costs, which at 22% appear to offer considerable scope for savings, are a particular target in the US (Etzioni, 1991, p.91). Fuchs (1990, p.538) suggests that a 'large one-time gain might be achieved by simplifying our [US] system of finance and reimbursement', pointing to Canada's large advantage with their physicians billing only one payer and hospitals not having to bill at all as they are 'paid according to a global annual budget'. Even the NHS, with its traditionally low administrative costs, is having to recognise that the 1991 changes greatly increased transaction costs and it is not yet proven whether or not these costs will be reduced with the implementation of the proposals in *The New NHS* (DoH, 1997).

Elimination of non-effective treatments

It is argued that there would be no, or less, need to ration beneficial treatments if all ineffective or non-beneficial treatments, all unnecessary treatments and all those treatments which actually do harm were eliminated. Few could object to the discontinuing of treatments which are proved to be harmful or of no benefit. Clearly the elimination of such treatments must be beneficial and would at the very least relieve pressure on the provision of beneficial treatments. However, in practice it is not so simple. Few treatments are never harmful and there are few treatments which never give any benefit at all to any patient (Jennett, 1988, p.98). Despite the current promotion of evidence-based medicine (EBM), for many procedures the evidence does not, and may not ever, exist in the rigorous form required by the advocates of EBM. And, as Weale (1995a, p.835) points out, 'it would be difficult to maintain the view that all untested medical procedures are guilty until proven innocent'. Nevertheless, Roberts *et al.* (1995b) suggest that 30% of current services do not stand up to their 'criteria of rationality', which include measurement of clinical effectiveness. However, what constitutes unnecessary, and possibly even non-effective, treatment is not solely the province of technical or clinical judgement but can also involve values. Further, health authorities have found great difficulty in eliminating services whose effectiveness is questionable. The public too may well take the stance that something is better than nothing.

There are claims that some instances of 'rationing' merely constitute the non-supply of non-beneficial treatments (Hunt, 1995). Clearly, on most of the definitions of rationing offered above, the denial of proven non-effective or non-beneficial treatment does not constitute rationing.

So, is it necessary to ration healthcare?

A rather pessimistic or defeatist thread can be detected running through a number of arguments. Starting from the notion that demand/need will always outstrip supply, it argues that, since greater efficiency, increased resource allocation, reduction of waste and elimination of totally ineffective treatments would not individually (or even combined) eliminate the need for rationing (in some form or another), they are either not worth pursuing or should be relegated to a secondary position behind the 'hard choices' of explicit rationing. It may well be that no society can, or would wish to, provide absolutely every medical intervention and form of care that are conceivably possible (but not necessarily needed or even demanded). However, rationing/priority setting in the presence of a generous resource allocation is likely to be far less painful – will need fewer 'hard choices' – than rationing/priority setting in the face of severely constrained resources.

Should healthcare be rationed?

If the argument is accepted that rationing is necessary or inevitable because it will never be possible to provide sufficient resources to meet need/demand, it may seem unnecessary to debate whether or not healthcare *should* be rationed. If, however, it is conceded that the inevitability of rationing is at least debatable, it is worth turning to some of the ethical and practical problems raised by rationing. Some general points will be considered here, whilst problems raised by some specific approaches to rationing and priority setting will be discussed in Chapter 4.

Detraction from underfunding

In contrast to the argument that rationing would be unnecessary or, at least, less severe if the NHS were better funded, Hunter (1993a, p.24) suggests that 'explicit rationing could divert attention from a basic under-funding of provision'. There is already a tendency within the post-1991 NHS to assume that additional expenditure on one healthcare service must automatically be at the expense of other healthcare services. This view is understandable, in the short term at least, for an individual purchaser attempting to allocate its fixed budget. However, to follow the question 'Is the public willing to forgo £190 million of general NHS services, the expenditure of one to two medium sized District General Hospitals, to provide the drug [β-interferon] for even one half of the 38,000 MS sufferers in the UK with the relapsing and remitting form of the disease?' with the statement 'The public debate must be made in the context of opportunity cost rather than the provision of extra resources' (Zimmern, 1995, p.9) would appear to fuel Hunter's fears that explicit rationing 'could blunt arguments for devoting additional resources to health care'.

A variant on assuming the total NHS resource to be fixed and unchangeable and accepting that any new developments must be at the expense of other NHS activities is 'rationing by budget'. This is illustrated in the increasing tendency to present, and possibly demonstrate the unaffordability of, new developments in terms of their impact on the particular budget-head under which they fall. For example, Walley and Barton

(1995, p.797) estimate that if 45% of the 85 000 multiple sclerosis patients were to receive interferon-β, the annual cost would be £380 million which, they note, is about 10% of the entire national drug bill. However, it is this latter point, rather than the careful discussion and proposals which surround it, that is cited by those who argue the inevitability of rationing. Taken to its logical conclusion, this approach would mean that even cost-saving innovations would not be implemented if the costs fell on one budget-head and the savings accrued to another.

Detraction from efficiency

It can also be claimed that the rationing debate serves as a diversion from questions of efficiency and the cost of delivering care. If rationing is taken as axiomatic, might there be less incentive to seek cost reductions and the removal of inefficiencies? In the post-1991 NHS the 'efficiency' savings and price reductions, forced on providers by purchasers, might have served to mitigate this danger. However, the increasing specificity and detail encouraged in contracts between purchasers and providers (a necessary pre-condition of explicit rationing?) may be costly in the fragmentation of what are essentially joint products. It remains to be seen whether the proposed service agreements (DoH, 1997) will perpetuate this trend.

Social justice

Arguments for rationing are often put forward in the name of social justice, on the analogy of the rationing of food during and after the last war or petrol rationing during a fuel crisis. Such rationing aims to secure fair shares for all, rather than letting the price of a scarce commodity rise and allowing the rich to purchase as much as they want and denying any to the poor. However, for this analogy to hold within healthcare, it would be necessary to forbid anyone to purchase care which is excluded from those who are rationed. Otherwise, rationing healthcare 'merely extends the prevailing class structure to health care' (Etzioni, 1991, p.94). Or, as other US commentators express it, 'If ... we allow some individuals to purchase the otherwise excluded medically necessary procedure, it would appear that we are restricting access based on ability to pay rather than on the category of illness' (Nelson and Drought, 1992, p.103).

Hadorn and Brook (1991, p.3328), quoting a dictionary definition of rationing as 'equitable distribution of scarce items, often necessities, by a system that limits individual portions', suggest that the World War II analogy applies only to organ transplantation and intensive care beds, where there is genuine scarcity. They go on to suggest that currently, far from fairness, rationing has come to represent discrimination.

As observed earlier, most advocates of healthcare rationing focus on publicly funded healthcare. Although it will be recalled that some commentators defined rationing as denying access to services, even to those willing and able to pay (Aaron, 1992; Pawlson *et al.*, 1992), there appear to be few people actually advocating this type of rationing. For instance, Nelson and Drought (1992, p.104), quoted above, suggest that there 'is no compelling reason why an individual should not be allowed to use his own private resources to purchase medical care above and beyond the established basic level of benefits'. However, Aaron and Schwartz (1990, p.418) devote an article to the question of 'whether health care should be rationed in this sense, whether its availability should be limited, even to those who can pay for it'. In a fascinating article on the Norwegian health service, Norheim (1995) draws on a wide range of ethical, social and practical arguments in his consideration of whether it is ethically justifiable to forbid people to purchase beneficial healthcare which has been excluded from the publicly funded healthcare system.

Rationing versus quality

Should the possibility of trading quality for quantity be offered? This may seem a curious point but, since its inception, it would appear that one reason why the NHS delivered a relatively large amount of healthcare for, by international standards, a relatively low share of GDP was that lower quality was accepted in non-clinical areas (e.g. long waits, shabby buildings, restricted choice). Without condoning long waits and poor amenities, it is worth noting that quality improvements are not automatically costless and, in the absence of an increase in resources, may result in a reduction in the quantity of treatment available. For instance, provided inefficiencies have been removed, shorter waiting times can be guaranteed only at the expense of numbers treated (Mullen, 1994). The ACHCEW (1993, p.22) Briefing quotes South Manchester HA as stating that the 'requirement to contain waiting times for in-patient admission within specific limits, given the resource position, means that it is not possible to accept all the referrals that are received'. Returning to the five Ds, perhaps if the public are to be consulted about priorities, they should be given an opportunity to express a view on Delay as an alternative to Denial. In many ways, centrally driven initiatives on waiting lists actually prevent the public from engaging in a discussion of this option.

On a totally different level, the Oregon plan can be seen as an attempt to spread very high-quality (in both clinical and non-clinical aspects) services more thinly over the non-insured population. The alternative of spreading rather lower quality services rather more thickly was not really considered, especially as providers were assured that their reimbursement levels would not be reduced (Brannigan, 1993). However, Veatch (1992, p.88), commenting on Oregon, suggests that:

The real issue is not whether to perform the appendectomy; it is whether to fund countless marginal interventions that are potentially part of the procedure – marginal blood tests and repeat tests; precautionary, preventive antibiotic therapy before surgery; the number of nurses in the operating room; and the backup support on call or in the hospital.

Should Dilution be considered as a positive alternative to Denial? Indeed, the Swedish Parliamentary Priorities Commission (1995, p.107) suggests that, in certain situations, 'it may be reasonable to opt for the second best treatment' in the face of limited resources.

Weale (1998, p.410) suggests that the basic principle of the NHS 'that comprehensive, high quality medical care should be [freely] available to all citizens' threatens to become 'an inconsistent triad'. Perhaps, he suggests, we can have any two of these propositions but at the expense of the third; for instance, 'a comprehensive service freely available to all, but not of high quality'. Each pair of propositions selected at the expense of the third 'defines a characteristic position in the modern debate about healthcare costs and organisation' and is, Weale demonstrates, associated with a range of 'problems'. Such value conflicts, he concludes, are the essence of public policy.

If the public are to be consulted about priorities, should they not also be asked their views on quantity versus quality (Denial v Dilution or Delay)? If rationing, in the form of denial, is too readily accepted as inevitable, this question may never be considered.

Limits to rationing

The fact that rationing can be applied only to some aspects of healthcare introduces a distortion. Some care must be given; for example, some emergency treatment, treatment of fractures, etc. In addition, there is a strong pre-supposition in favour of continuing treatment once started, regardless of the cost/benefit calculus at later points in the treatment; for example, the treatment of endstage renal failure (ESRF). Thus protocols and exclusions could result in two patients with identical conditions and currently identical circumstances, one receiving treatment and the other being refused, merely because the first patient was, say, younger at the onset of their illness. These factors not only restrict the range of treatment and care which can be subject to the rationing process but also limit the 'rationality' of the whole procedure.

So, should healthcare be rationed?

Thus, not only is it argued that it may not be necessary to ration healthcare, it is argued that unquestioning acceptance of the necessity or inevitability of rationing is self-defeating. Not only does it raise ethical problems but acceptance of the need for rationing can distract us from attempting to remove or alleviate the perceived causes of that rationing. Further, the macho tendency in the debate, stressing the need for 'hard choices' and focusing on denial, not only raises the emotional temperature of the debate but detracts from the many other areas where choices must be made in delivering healthcare services and where priority setting is essential.

CHAPTER THREE

Consumer involvement in healthcare

Why consumer involvement?

Although the current interest in involving consumers in healthcare is often attributed to the publication of *Local Voices* (DoH, 1992), consumer participation in health has a long, if somewhat patchy, history (Toth, 1996). The 1970s in particular saw an upsurge of interest in consumer participation, not only in the UK but in many developed countries. For instance, in the United States various Acts passed during the 1970s called for a greater role in health planning by consumers of healthcare and in some cases these Acts specifically defined and required consumer participation (Cooper, 1979; Koseki, 1977). In Italy, Modolo and Figa-Talamanca (1977, p.41) reported that:

> in the last few years professionals at all levels have become increasingly aware of the need to involve the population in the planning and carrying out of health programmes. We have thus been witnessing a change in the relationship between the health worker and the community . . .

In a review of USA and western European literature, Van Den Heuval (1980, p.423) stated that the 'idea of involving the "consumer" in (the) "health-industry" has become widely accepted', but he added that this was not 'without resistance from providers and planners'.

Many commentators located this increased interest in, and demand for, consumer participation in the general increase in 'consumerism' observed in the late 1960s and 1970s. Christensen and Wertheimer (1976, p.406) argued that:

> The contemporary demand by consumers for community participation and control may be viewed as a logical response to a perceived growing impersonalism and lack of responsiveness of large governmental and social service systems.

In respect of social services, George and Wilding (1985, p.143) suggest that since the early 1970s important sections of the public in many welfare capitalist societies have been critical of the organisational structures of social services, citing 'their private and undemocratic decision-making processes, their unresponsiveness to consumer convenience and to public complaints and their over-reliance on professional experts'. This, they claim, 'has led to demands for greater public participation in the management and organisation of social services'.

However, Christensen and Wertheimer (1976) and other commentators suggested that there were special factors relating to health and healthcare which contributed to the increasing demands for participation. They suggested that, as consumers became better educated and more sophisticated about healthcare, their growing expectations contrasted with the substantial problems related to the delivery of medical care. Within the American context, Kelman (1976, p.431) saw the increasing acceptance of consumer involvement in health services planning, organisation and delivery 'as a necessary and important concomitant of efforts designed to refashion our "crisis-ridden" health care system'.

Van Den Heuval (1980, p.423) stated that the:

professional domination of the healthcare system is followed by a bureaucratic one . . . (which) promotes the economic concepts of supply and demand; patients are consumers of health industry. At the same time movements on human rights, self-care and individual responsibility ask for availability of adequate medical care, for human care and patient rights; patients are independent and critical consumers.

Mishra (1984, p.128) takes this further, stating that 'social policy is manipulated by the professions manning the service to their own advantage. This seems to be one of the features of the development of social services within a capitalist society. . .'. He observes that 'the development of the social services has led to greater centralisation and bureaucratisation; this has meant a decline in the power of lay interests, for example the friendly societies and other voluntary organisations'. This process, he argues, does not have to result in a concentration of power in the hands of professionals and administrators. The main reason there is such a concentration of power, he suggests, is:

that the growth of professionalism and the wresting of control from lay hands has not been followed by any substantive (i.e. more than token) attempt to give countervailing power to the consumers. Thus what seems to have happened is a net transfer of power to the professionals . . .

George and Wilding (1985, p.143) suggest that arguments of both principle and practice support the case for participation.

The argument of principle is obvious – services for people in a democratic society should involve citizens directly in their running. The argument of practice is that services will be more effective if geared directly to the needs expressed by actual or potential users rather than being based on decisions made by professionals and bureaucrats.

Thus the highest level of argument for involving the public in priority setting is centred upon the notion of democracy in society, the rights and responsibilities of citizenship and the issue of democratic accountability on the part of health authorities.

Calnan (1995, p.18), however, makes a clear distinction between citizen views and user views, arguing that taking the former into account 'may serve as a means of democratising health services, thus making both the medical profession and the state more accountable'. He suggests four reasons why user views should be heeded. First, the emphasis on quality of healthcare means that measures of social acceptability to users should count alongside clinical and economic measures in healthcare evaluation. Second, with the shift from acute to chronic diseases, 'sufferers and their families play a more active part in management'. Third, patient satisfaction may increase 'compliance' with treatment. Finally, he cites humanitarian concerns – 'the altruistic concern of the doctor with the users' welfare' – especially related to the holistic view of care and the ethical concern which emphasises 'the need to inform patients about the risks of different treatments', leaving the decision to them.

Lomas (1997) articulates the complexity of the issues relating to public involvement. He suggests that each individual (adult) exists in multiple roles as he/she is asked to engage in the decision-making process. An individual may well be a taxpayer with an interest in the total amount of money allocated to health services. The same person may well at some stage be a recipient of healthcare services in one form or another and therefore interested in the experience of healthcare. Finally, the individual is located in a particular area of the country and will have views about the provision and pattern of local services. It is very likely that views expressed within each of these roles separately will be in conflict.

However, it is important to note that representative democracy, via the ballot box, is usually considered to be the 'correct' route for citizen participation.* Coote (1993, p.38) argues that, in theory at least, it 'addresses the diverse and shared interests of the population as a whole'. Of course, in the case of the NHS, elected authority resides only at the national level and not at the local level. However, even in respect of social services, George and Wilding (1985, p.143) suggest that 'Management, through the normal processes of local government, does not guarantee appropriate democratic control'. Coote (1993, p.38) argues that 'in a large and complex society, the distances between the decision and the representative, and between the representative and the elector are so great that the amount of power actually exercised by the individual citizen is negligible'. Hill and Bramley (1986, pp.203–4) sum up the arguments of many commentators:

Modern arguments for participation rest on a view that the right to vote is not enough, a view that in a complex society in which complex policies are formulated and implemented other modes of citizen intervention are necessary. There is an analytical problem, therefore, about what is implied by participation. A claim to participate is a claim to be given more power ...

---

* Indeed, some members of an international audience professed to be baffled by the UK pursuit of public involvement in healthcare priority setting, suggesting that it should be the role of the elected authorities.

Nevertheless, the claim of representative democracy to be the most – the only – legitimate form of participation cannot be ignored. The interest within the NHS in consulting the public at local level could, on the one hand, be viewed sympathetically as an attempt to compensate for the lack of elected democratic control at local level but, on the other hand, it could be viewed as an attempt to distract attention from the lack of such control.[*]

The role of the consumer in healthcare

Apart from the argument, put forward by Doll (1979) and others, that the proper role of individual consumers is to take more care of their own health, there are many different roles ascribed to the consumer or to consumer participation. These include: the education of consumers; advocacy of patients' rights/dealing with individual complaints (Gosfield, 1976); self-help (which often contains a degree of antiprofessionalism, antitechnology and alternative medicine) (Hatch, 1978); influencing the priorities and direction of the healthcare system/participation in planning (Van Den Heuval, 1980).

Types of consumer involvement

The extent and type of consumer involvement in healthcare vary considerably (Feuerstein, 1980). Arnstein (1969, 1971) demonstrates this in her useful 'ladder of participation' (Box 3.1), which descends from citizen control, through consultation and informing, to manipulation.

Box 3.1:   Arnstein's ladder of citizen participation (Arnstein, 1969, 1971)

Citizen control
Delegated power
Partnership
Placation
Consultation
Informing
Therapy
Manipulation

Mullen *et al.* (1982, 1984) made a distinction between 'reactive' consumer involvement and '(pro-)active' or 'initiator' involvement. This distinction affects not only the

---

[*] See Pollock (1992) for a useful discussion of these issues.

mechanisms used to secure involvement but also the view that is taken of the function, validity and very nature of consumer involvement by the provider and by society. In the former case, the role of the consumer is to *react* to activities, plans, proposals and priorities that emanate from within the healthcare system. Mechanisms by which this type of consumer involvement is secured include consultation with consumer organisations or consumer representatives and the conducting of consumer opinion or satisfaction surveys.

With both consultation and consumer surveys, the 'framework' within which the decisions are made – within which the services are planned or delivered – is formulated by the professionals or managers and there is little scope for consumer influence. To a large extent, the values and priorities incorporated in the proposals offered for consultation, or in the survey questions, are also those of the professionals or managers. Further, unless the consultation or surveys are carried out at an extremely early stage in the decision-making process, there is a very real risk that many of the original options will have been closed before there is any possibility of consumer influence (Dunford, 1977).

Equating consumer involvement with consumer reaction can betray the professional's view of the consumer. Kelman (1976, p.433), referring specifically to consumer involvement in the evaluation of healthcare quality, argues that some professionals and managers tend to regard consumers, or 'recipients' of care, essentially as data sources, often within studies where the parameters being measured 'are not necessarily the *dimensions* of major concern to consumers'. Locker and Dunt (1978, p.290) add to this point, stating that true studies of consumer evaluation 'would need to identify and employ criteria for standards used by consumers themselves'. Van Den Heuval (1980, p.425) states that:

> most research on evaluation and satisfaction of consumers in health care analyses socio-cultural and socio-economic variables and experiences in health/illness. They are less useful for establishing the position of the consumer in health care or in contributing to an increase in the influence of consumer opinion in health policy.

'Active' or 'initiator' involvement, in contrast, requires that consumers have more influence on proposals, especially on their initiation and formulation. One mechanism, which is often proposed to effect this type of involvement, is consumer participation in the decision-making or management bodies themselves. However, whilst this could, in theory, overcome many of the problems outlined above, it is not without its drawbacks. Paap (1978, p.578) identifies structural problems relating to language, organisation of meetings, exclusion from information channels, ambiguity of role, etc. which inhibit any effective consumer control even where consumers form the majority of the decision-making bodies and which 'thereby perpetuate the traditional power structure of providers and other professionals in the health care fields'.

On the other hand, there is the fear that consumer or public representatives on decision-making bodies will become 'incorporated', moving away from their constituency and becoming indistinguishable from the professionals and managers; 'participants become unrepresentative through their participation' (Richardson, 1983, p.65). Similar risks may face standing panels of consumers or the now frequently advocated 'citizens' juries' (Lenaghan, 1996b; Lenaghan *et al.*, 1997; Stewart *et al.*, 1994), where the lay participants have long-term and/or intensive exposure to professional and managerial views.

Hogwood and Gunn (1984, p.115) identify issue definition as the policy process stage where:

> *there is a particularly strong case for wider participation by those in a position to say whether there is a problem and, if so, what they see the problem as being. In practice opportunities for participation tend to be provided, if at all, only at the later stages of the policy process, such as commenting on 'options' provided by officials. By then most real choices will have been foreclosed, whereas an opportunity to participate in how the problem was defined would have opened up a much wider range of possibilities . . .*

However, it must be noted that, as the methods necessary to secure proactive participation are usually far more demanding on the public than are reactive methods, there is a risk of bias. Johnson *et al.* (1993), writing about public participation in wildlife management, found that those attending public meetings exhibited different characteristics and had different views from a similar number of randomly selected people completing questionnaires. Coote (1993) also discusses the problems of representativeness associated with the more active forms of participation.

Hill and Bramley (1986, pp.202–3) take a more fundamental line, suggesting that the way participation is viewed depends on the way the evolution of welfare policy is explained. They identify three categories of explanation. The first sees 'welfare policies as essentially social control policies advanced by dominant elites reluctant to share economic or political power' and thus views participation as 'essentially palliative . . . designed to damp down conflict whilst not conceding power'. The second views welfare policies 'as the product of concern by elites about inequalities and human suffering' and thus 'those with power and responsibility will be seen as exercising them responsively, and devices to enhance participation will be seen as largely unnecessary . . . [as] . . . those delivering benefits and services should be trusted to operate in the best interests of their clients'. According to this explanation, participation is 'seen as getting in the way of the smooth operation of the policy'. The third group of explanations sees welfare policies as responses to democratic political demands and thus offers 'approaches which can most easily find a place for the participative devices . . . Forms of participation, particularly when organised through pressure groups, are seen as a significant political force . . .'

Legitimising decisions

Involving the public in determining priorities for the rationing of services can serve to legitimise those decisions. Ham (1993, p.436) sees this as an advantage, stating that:

The process of setting priorities involves making judgements on the basis of incomplete information and evidence. These judgements are likely to be more soundly based and defensible if they have been exposed to public discussion.

However, Hunter (1993a, p.27) voices the concern 'that many of those championing public involvement are not in fact seeking to empower people in order to enable them to participate effectively but rather may be seeking a superficial legitimacy – a veneer – for management decisions about priorities'. This could be argued to constitute a misuse of public participation since incorporating the public in the decision-making process undermines their ability to challenge the whole notion of priority setting as well as deflecting criticism of the actual priority decisions. To take a somewhat cynical perspective, it is perhaps not surprising that the upsurge in interest in public consultation should coincide with the concern of most societies to curb expenditure on health systems. The objective of sharing the pain of difficult decisions has already been mentioned as one of the more calculated reasons for public involvement. However, purchasers wishing to use public participation in order to legitimise the denial of treatment or services might attempt to draw on the argument of prior consent.

Prior consent

Fleck (1992, p.1621) argues that 'Any fair approach to healthcare rationing must be a product of patient choice, freely and rationally self-imposed ...'. He further argues that:

If all who will be affected by rationing decisions have a fair opportunity to shape these decisions, then these rationing decisions will be freely self-imposed, which is an essential feature of just rationing decisions. (Fleck, 1994b, p.375)

At the level of the individual, it is argued that people should have the right to choose to subscribe to health plans which give restricted coverage and that 'general rationing rules and incentives can be disclosed to subscribers to health maintenance organizations (HMOs) and other limited insurance plans at the time of enrollment' (Hall, 1993, p.646). However, it can be questioned how freely consent to the restrictions is given, because of both lack of understanding and choice constraints at the time of enrolment (Appelbaum, 1993; Hall, 1994).

The prior consent argument then moves on to group decisions. Fleck (1992, p.1617) argues that 'If we can create public and social processes through which rationing decisions become something we collectively impose upon ourselves, then we will have rationing decisions that will have at least *prima facie* moral legitimacy'. He goes on to give the hypothetical example of a pool of 1000 women who, in order to control insurance premiums, agree amongst themselves to purchase screening mammograms, instead of providing autologous bone marrow transplants (ABMT) to those who develop cancer and need such treatment. Having benefited economically from the original decision, it would then be unjust for a member of this group, who subsequently develops endstage breast cancer, to attempt to secure ABMT for herself.

Group agreement to rationing raises difficult questions, many of which are relevant to discussions about priority setting in the NHS. Who makes the rationing decisions? How freely are they made? Can the group majority over-ride the views of the minority? How much choice do individuals have in their own membership of a group? It is argued that the Oregon exercise failed on the prior consent requirement because the poor, who are the main group affected, were largely excluded from the decision making (Nelson and Drought, 1992).

Fleck (1994b, p.381) claims that 'democracy is about respecting expressed preferences'. He discusses possible systems for democratic consensus which might be applicable in the presence of a single comprehensive health plan for the whole of society (Fleck, 1992). Writing later (1994a, p.441), he discusses rationing protocols 'freely and democratically chosen by the members of a given AHP [Accountable Health Plan]'. However, with the demise of the Clinton proposals, Fleck (1995a) sees the future for democratic consensus as being within managed care plans operating under global budgets.

In addition to being a response to *Local Voices* (DoH, 1992), is the current NHS interest in consulting the public on priority setting at the local level prompted by notions of prior consent? If it is, this must be viewed with some concern. The prior consent 'justification' is predicated on the individual, individually, agreeing to accept future restrictions on services. However, except for those services purchased by GPFHs, individuals could not, without moving house, select their purchaser. Even the Healthcare 2000 (1995) report, which advocated purchaser competition by ceasing to base health commissions on geographical areas, suggested that 'subscription' to health commissions could be based on employment or trade union membership and not individual subscription. Primary care groups (DoH, 1997) may potentially give individuals the opportunity to 'select their health plan' and thus give their (implied?) prior consent to any restrictions in access to services, provided such restrictions are made clear at the time of registration.

Of course, a range of other problems would arise if each individual could select their 'purchaser'. With increasing genetic knowledge of predisposition to illness, coupled with knowledge of pre-existing illnesses, the twin problems of cream skimming and adverse selection may prove insurmountable. The probability of devising 'a sophisticated system of allocating resources based on an actuarial assessment of risk of each individual member of the population' (Healthcare 2000, 1995, p.48) is near zero and, even if it were possible, it could itself lead to an interesting range of perverse incentives.

Whether or not such problems could be resolved, it would appear to be stretching the prior consent justification too far to suggest that the majority views of those members (even a representative sample) of the public (or 'health plan') consulted can be taken to imply prior consent by that community to restrictions on services or treatments.

Legitimacy of participation

In addition to fears that consumer involvement or participation in health and other public services may serve to legitimise managerial decisions, the notion of consumer involvement and participation itself raises a whole range of legitimacy issues.

Direct versus indirect participation and representativeness

First, there is the question posed by indirect consumer involvement, which arises in any area in respect of any services. Some commentators sidestep this by questioning whether there should be any indirect participation. Modolo and Figa-Talamanca (1977, p.42) state that 'The people involved should act in the first person, without delegating their rights and powers to representatives'.

However, since this is usually impractical, we return to the problem of the legitimacy or representativeness of consumers involved in participative processes. Are representatives only legitimised when they are elected? Do those involved have to be 'representative', i.e. typical of their constituency? How can it be ensured that the interests of minority groups are not overlooked? Should spokespeople for minority groups be involved and what is their legitimacy? Should the 'general public' be involved or only those in receipt of the particular service, i.e. should people participate as 'citizens' or as 'users' (Calnan, 1995)? Do the 'most vocal advocates have personal political goals' and do they therefore not 'represent the individual consumer's interest' (Gosfield, 1976, p.405)? Clearly there is considerable scope for debate here. Lomas (1997, p.105) observes that:

> The complexity arises from the observation that there is not necessarily any logical consistency in the preferences expressed independently in each of these domains. So that in our role as taxpayer we may oppose increased funding, whilst in our role of patient we may demand new and expensive services although in our role as local citizen we may oppose the exclusion of these same services being purchased on our behalf.

In addition, the problem of representing the individual experience, whether actual or imagined, in terms of perceptions about healthcare is virtually impossible in any statistical sense. The concept of average views or consensus views clearly disenfranchises potentially large minorities who have strong views about particular services.

However, there is still the question of the legitimacy of majority decision making and the issue of individual rights versus the collective; 'collective' decision making does 'not take seriously the individual right to access to health care based on need' (Doyal, 1993, p.50). It is not solely a question of the representativeness of those participating since the right of the majority to exclude some individuals, or whole groups, from receiving some service could be challenged even if there were 100% participation in decision making. This position can be characterised as anti-democratic but its proponents would counter with the risk of the dictatorship of the majority or 'an apparent tyranny of communal preferences over individual interest' (Brannigan, 1993, p.29).

But even if these questions were resolved, in theory, to the satisfaction of those concerned, it can be complex and costly actually to secure a representative group (Cooper, 1979). As will be discussed later, the practical importance of this issue will be affected by the nature of the decisions being made.

Consumers versus professionals

The second question of legitimacy is more specific to the area of health, although it also arises in related areas where there is a strong professional component. This is the question of whether the consumer, the layperson, citizens or the community as a whole have any legitimate role in assessing services, in planning healthcare or in determining priorities. Is there a risk of a 'dictatorship of the uninformed' (Hunter, 1993a, pp.18–19)? Kelman (1976, p.432) points out that 'Such activities on the part of consumers can be viewed as illegitimate intrusion into professional prerogatives' and that some professionals consider that only knowledgeable peers may make judgements of performance, leaving little or no room for consumers. However, Kelman goes on to argue that any exclusion of, or constraint on, consumer participation 'on the grounds of ignorance or incompetence is essentially an ideological denial of legitimacy'.

Jonas (1978) takes up this point, stating that 'A professional degree does not guarantee the ability to produce a programme beneficial to the people it serves' and Modolo and Figa-Talamanca (1977, p.42) go even further to argue that the professional (scientific) approach is not sufficient and that their experience had shown 'that the subjective approach, i.e. the judgement of the people, is even more important for planning health services'.*

The biomedical basis of most medical training, whereby illness is tackled by the application of specialist knowledge, has resulted in the practice of a benevolent paternalism.

> *Doctors have always emphasised the importance of authority in their relationship with their patients and based their own claim to clinical authority, the right to make decisions on the patients' behalf, on that authority.* (Faulder, 1985, p.24)

The implicit hierarchy between the various medical specialisms and the value placed on acute, high-technology based interventions bolster the notion that the general public cannot understand such complexities and that any involvement must therefore be at the margin of healthcare decision making.

Concern about participation by uninformed or ill-informed consumers has led, as will be discussed in Chapter Five, to methodologies such as citizens' juries, which attempt to ensure 'informed' participation by providing participants with information

---

* See Koseki (1977, pp.58–9) for further discussion of legitimacy.

prior to eliciting their views. However, although undoubtedly there are situations where consumer views, having been informed by the professionals, are appropriate, in other situations 'uncontaminated' views of consumers may be more relevant.

However, it has been suggested that consumer or public – but not professional – responses may be influenced by whether or not the respondent has experience of the condition or health state under consideration or by the probability of the respondent ever getting that condition (Menzel, 1992), i.e. the Rawlsian 'veil of ignorance' is absent. This latter effect might be particularly evident for congenital and early-onset conditions, which respondents know they will never experience personally.

Public attitudes may also be affected by the way in which health outcomes are viewed, since this depends upon an interaction between psychological and biological processes (Hyland, 1992). The psychological model emphasises the 'gap' between the attainment and aspiration related to particular goals. Health (or ill health) can be defined as the inability to attain once-expressed goals. Equally, goals can change or be redefined and some would argue psychological health can be expressed as the ability successfully to reinterpret goals following ill health.

Physical limitation and emotional distress can be viewed as different kinds of discontent attaching to the value of treatments or interventions. Thus a range of values may be placed on different kinds of health status and there is evidence of wide variation in this value judgement (McGee *et al.*, 1991).

Many health status or quality-of-life measures have been developed and even those that are multiattribute and patient oriented have as an underlying value a concern to capture what the patient regards as unsatisfactory or deficient in their condition. They thus represent a dominant value system and fail to incorporate the psychological restructuring of health states.

These different value perspectives have an important implication for public involvement in priority setting since the averaging of value measures maintains a dominant value set and, furthermore, masks major individual differences in conceptions of health status.

McIver (1997) also notes the problem of obtaining clear views about service provision from individuals who have no experience of it. This is linked to the vulnerability of various methods of obtaining public views (surveys and opinion polls) which offer limited degrees of dialogue with the public. Finally, on a slightly depressing note for advocates of public involvement, Lomas (1997, p.108) concludes: 'If the objective of involving citizens in rationing is to allocate resources cost effectively within a constrained budget and improve equity within the system, then using the general public as the determining voice appears unlikely to contribute'.

The problem also arises of what to do when public/lay and professional views differ, especially when the public give, in the view of the professionals, the 'wrong' answers, e.g. rating intensive care for premature babies higher than hip joint replacements (Bowling, 1993, p.54). Whose views or values should prevail?

Some who caution against moving from an implicit to a more explicit approach to allocating health service resources may be motivated by either (a) the threat that implicit rationing, the appropriate preserve of the professional, will be taken away, with associated loss of power and control or (b) the genuine concern that due to either weakness in methodologies employed or the complexities of the content, the public are unable to enter the debate in a meaningful way.

This somewhat elitist perspective may be reinforced by the current conflicts surrounding the NHS's attempts to rationalise and centralise services into larger but fewer hospital sites. Vociferous public support for local A&E (accident and emergency) units and for the preservation of small local hospitals may be seen as uninformed and counter to the increasingly shared professional view that better clinical outcomes will result from grouping services together on a single site.

However, this argument may simply suggest that the public cannot play a meaningful role when they do not have the appropriate information. The issue then moves to one of process, of how such information should be disseminated. If this process is successfully undertaken but the public still express views counter to those of professional opinion we then face the real crux of the debate on public involvement in priority setting. Is the public being asked to make the decision or is it taking part in a process where other views, probably professional views, will be given greater weight in the final decision?

Populism

Pateman (1970, p.1) gives a rather different view of legitimacy. She finds it rather ironic that participation should have become so popular since, she argues, 'the concept of participation has only the most minimal role in the theory of democracy widely accepted by political theorists and political sociologists'. They would place emphasis 'on the dangers inherent in wide popular participation in politics'. She goes on to report (p.3) that 'large-scale empirical investigations into political attitudes have revealed ... that widespread non-democratic or authoritarian attitudes exist'. Thus, she suggests, 'an increase in political participation by present non-participants could upset the stability of the democratic system'. Fears of such populism could lead to worries that the public may indulge in 'victim blaming' or downgrade unpopular diseases.

Inevitably, there is a fear that the public, whether through prejudice, preconceptions or misconceptions, will downgrade the importance given to unpopular, less glamorous conditions (mental illness and disability) or where some blame might be said to attach to the victim, e.g. AIDS (Harrison and Hunter, 1994; Robinson, 1997). In a similar vein, Bowling *et al.* (1993, p.856) concluded a study of priority setting in a disadvantaged area of London by saying:

> *Priorities based on community perceptions alone might be contrary to the spirit of equity and equal access according to need which is still espoused as a central philosophy of the NHS. The lower value placed on mental health and the elderly of the public in this study compared to providers, underlines this concern.*

Power and professional resistance

A further problem that arises with consumer participation is that it can encounter resistance from the professionals or can even lead to open conflict between consumers and providers. This can arise, Kelman (1976, p.431) claims, because 'the more or less exclusive prerogative that the provider group enjoyed in decision-making in health is to be shared, to a greater or lesser degree, with consumers, their representatives, or persons acting on their behalf' or as Koseki (1977, p.55) puts it, rather more strongly, 'the prime issue in consumer participation is one of sharing power'. Further, Paap and Hanson (1979, p.179) point out that the concept of consumer-based boards (to control health centres in the USA) is 'founded on the view that consumers and professionals have different interests'. George and Wilding (1985, p.144) point out that 'Securing participation means major and radical changes in the ethos and structure of service' and thus it will be opposed 'by those whose convenience and interests are threatened by its introduction and implications . . .'.

The control of power by professionals or providers can itself inhibit true participation. Johnson (1974, p.90) points out that professional interests control information and that since 'The hospital or the District is to be seen not only as a therapeutic territory, but as a complex power arena in which different sorts of information play a vital part', it is difficult for a body external to the system to obtain the necessary materials to assemble policies. Paap (1978, p.581) claims that the bureaucratic style of meetings and functioning required by the organisation 'can have a negative impact on consumers' feeling about their competence'.

Recognising the growing influence of consumers, some health institutions, professionals and administrators have sought to deflect the challenge to their power. One way is to claim consumer participation as their own initiative and 'to work with the consumer and try to direct their influence into specific fields of, for example, "prevention" in which they stress people's "own responsibility"' (Van Den Heuval, 1980). This approach is neatly illustrated by Ast (1978, p.16) who states that 'Consumer power has a dominant role to play in promoting good health, habits and practices. Let us (i.e. professionals) learn to work effectively with it'. Another way to deflect the consumer challenge is for the professional interests to set things up in such a way that consumers will tend to concentrate on administrative details rather than on areas of policy formulation (Paap, 1978).

At the same time, almost as a mirror image, there is some evidence of resistance from the public to answering questions directed specifically at setting priorities for treatments and services (Dicker and Armstrong, 1995 *inter alia*) and also to answering 'willingness to pay' type questions. Several studies indicate that a majority of respondents consider that such decision making should be left to doctors and other experts (Bowling, 1993, p.43; Heginbotham, 1993, p.147; Richardson *et al.*, 1992).

One might also hypothesise that the public are aware of the uncomfortable nature of these decisions. Although some studies do report the public's willingness to prioritise services, it is at very high levels of generality such as 'nursing services', 'acute emergencies' or 'primary care' (Bowling *et al.*, 1993; Richardson *et al.*, 1992). On the whole, the evidence is that citizens do not want to take on the responsibility of being collective decision makers for their fellows. Abelson *et al.* (1995) report two-thirds of their Canadian sample did not want to take responsibility for priority setting. This is similar to the findings of Dicker and Armstrong (1995, p.1139) in the UK, who conclude: 'Overall these findings challenge the idea that local voices should have great prominence in decisions about resource allocations. These interviewees felt ill-equipped to become involved in the process'. The more specific the level of enquiry, the more difficult it seems to become. The New Zealand Core Services Committee also foundered on this in their attempt to define a core set of services (Cumming, 1994).

CHAPTER FOUR

Priority setting, rationing and the consumer role

As noted in Chapter Two, the broader and relatively neutral concept of priority setting has in recent years been overshadowed by the more narrowly focused rationing debate. The 'hard choices' of which treatments should and should not be supplied, which patients should or should not be treated, now commonly associated with rationing, do of course constitute an aspect of priority setting. However, there is a far wider range of issues relating to the NHS where choices have to be made, priorities need to be set and where preferences should be taken into account. These range from the national level where the decision is made as to what priority to give to the NHS as compared to the other competing claims for national public funds, through a range of issues such as centralising versus dispersing facilities, to the very local level where priorities are set in the way that services are delivered (e.g. what priority should be given to ensure the availability of female doctors) or the order in which they are delivered. Some of the areas which involve the setting of priorities, in one form or another, are indicated in Box 4.1.

Despite the fact that areas which relate to *how* services are provided are of profound importance to providers and users of health services, as well as the general public, they have been overshadowed in much of the recent debate by the questions of which services should be provided and to whom – explicit rationing. Thus, initially, some priority-setting approaches associated with explicit rationing will be examined, followed by consideration of public involvement in priority setting in general.

Box 4.1:   Some areas of priority setting in the NHS

- Between the NHS and other sectors
- Between competing values, e.g. rights v rewards
- In targeting diseases
- Between different treatments/services to be offered
- In how and where health services are to be provided
- Order of treatment (selection from waiting lists, A&E, etc.)
- In non-medical aspects (appointment systems, waiting, food, decor)
- Between different patient groups (old v young, men v women)
- In choice of treatment

Setting priorities according to health gain and QALY maximisation

Drawing on the assumption that the objective of the NHS is to maximise health, it is frequently argued that priority setting should focus on maximising health gain. Indeed, many commentators treat maximising health gain as being synonymous with healthcare rationing.

The primary tool associated with this approach is the quality-adjusted life year (QALY). Priorities are based on the cost per QALY, with the aim of maximising the number of QALYs obtained. QALY league tables have been produced ranking treatments in order of cost per QALY. On the face of it, this approach, which seeks to maximise benefit in terms of health gain achieved within available resources, appears both attractive and obvious. Indeed, Williams (1995, p.223) challenges the reader to consider whether, under the Rawlsian 'veil of ignorance', they 'would choose a set of rules which would maximise the health of the community as a whole, as measured in QALY terms, and, if not, why not?'. However, prioritisation by health gain and QALY maximisation have come under criticism from a number of directions.

Before examining these criticisms, it is worth noting that health gain approaches use other techniques as well as, and instead of, QALY maximisation. Many approaches start with the concept of needs assessment and use epidemiological methods to identify areas of unmet need (see Hunter (1993b) for discussion of health gain). Some such exercises give high priority weights to treatment for conditions which have the highest incidence or prevalence. This is somewhat difficult to understand. Although it is unarguable, *mutatis mutandis*, that more resources should be allocated to conditions affecting larger numbers of people, it does not follow that conditions should be given a higher priority merely because they affect a larger number of people. To argue that they should would effectively be to claim that the rarity of a disease is, in itself, justification for giving it low priority.

Construction of QALYs

Some criticisms of QALYs, and similar health status measures, relate to methodological problems in their construction and calibration, including how different levels and dimensions of quality of life are measured, how different health states are valued, how values are elicited (Carr-Hill, 1989), whose values should be used and what the resulting values mean (Nord, 1990). These are all very important issues for priority setting. For instance, these points are illustrated by controversy surrounding the initial draft list of conditions/treatment pairs in Oregon, which was based on cost-utility using the Quality of Well-Being (QWB) Scale. This list contained apparently counter-intuitive rankings (for example, ranking tooth capping above appendectomy), which were widely blamed on incomplete or inaccurate information (Kaplan, 1992). But Nord (1993) argues that the counter-intuitive rankings were caused by the unfounded assumption that QWB values have cardinal properties, whilst at the same time the methods used for eliciting values resulted in insufficient compression of values at the upper end of the scale, thus overvaluing small improvements in already fairly healthy people. However, Hadorn (1991b, p.2219) suggests that the rankings did not occur as the result of faulty data but 'as an inevitable consequence of the application of cost-effectiveness analysis'.

QALYs are also criticised for what their advocates claim is their main strength – the combining of quality of life with length of life and the resulting direct comparison (trade-off) of life-saving treatments with quality-enhancing treatments (Harris, 1987).

In addition, as noted in Chapter Three, many health status or quality-of-life measures capture what the patient regards as unsatisfactory or deficient in their condition, thus failing to incorporate the psychological restructuring of health states.

How quality-of-life scales are constructed, how values are elicited, whose values are used and what the resulting values mean are all important questions, some of which will be considered later. At this point the discussion on QALY maximisation will proceed on the (possibly very unreasonable) set of assumptions that an acceptable quality-of-life scale has been devised, that there is a satisfactory methodology for determining values and, with a few exceptions, there is general agreement on whose values should be used.

Equity

Maximising total health gain, without consideration of distributive effects, is essentially utilitarian and thus raises a range of ethical objections to utilitarianism, including those relating to individual justice and equity. The failure to incorporate equity issues is recognised by some advocates of QALYs, who stress that 'there will be a need for a purchasing authority to form a view about what weight it will attach to equity concerns relative to those of efficiency' (Mooney *et al.*, 1992, p.9). Maynard (1996b, p.1499) concedes that society 'may be prepared to forgo efficient health gains in order to behave "fairly"' but adds that if 'health gains are to be sacrificed to achieve fairness' both that concept must be defined and the resulting reduction in health gain monitored.

Equity in healthcare, itself, is not a simple concept; Harrison and Hunter (1994) suggest 18 definitions. However, a widely accepted view is that equity in healthcare implies the principle of equal access for equal need – itself not an unproblematic concept. It is claimed that the QALY maximisation or health gain approach violates this principle. As Lockwood (1988, p.45) puts it, the principle 'to each according to what will generate the most QALYs' is potentially in conflict with 'to each according to his need'. Rather than treating people with equal need equally, QALY maximisation will accord differential access to people with equal need for treatment, where the cost of treating them is different (Harris, 1988). Thus systematic discrimination could result against, say, those from ethnic minority groups who require interpreters, those living in poorer housing who might require inpatient stays rather than day surgery and those living in remote sparsely populated locations, etc. To take a hypothetical example, suppose there were a condition, suffered by both men and women, for which treatment gave equal health gain to both sexes but, for some biological reason, treatment for a woman costs far more than treatment for a man. Would it be acceptable to follow the logic of QALY maximisation and give treatment of men higher priority than treatment of women? If the answer is negative, the health gain maximisers would retort that treating women equally with men under such circumstances would result in greater overall suffering and less aggregate health gain or, more emotively, be 'expensive in terms of death and suffering' (Mooney, 1989, p.149).

Similar arguments could be made where people are in equal need but would achieve different levels of health gain from the same amount of resources and, possibly even more forcefully, where those in greater health need find themselves ranked as lower priority than those in less health need, because the cost per QALY of their treatment is greater.

Double jeopardy

Related to the equity argument is the claim that QALY maximisation may cause discrimination against people with a pre-existing disability because their potential QALY gain from, say, a particular life-saving treatment is inherently lower than the potential gain from the same treatment received by a person who can be restored to full health. Harris (1987, 1988) argues that this involves a form of double jeopardy. Because a person has already been a victim of a disaster resulting in a lower quality of life, QALYs rule them out (or give them lower priority) as a candidate for life-saving treatment.

Another argument relating to people with pre-existing disabilities, but which is somewhat outside the scope of the discussion here, arises in the valuing of the different health states. It is argued that there is potential for discrimination against the disabled if states of health are valued by those who have never experienced them.

Individual versus the collective and the 'rule of rescue'

The question of the individual versus the collective is possibly the most difficult issue associated with the maximisation of health gain. Not only does it raise a range of ethical issues, it also leads, as we shall see later, to practical difficulties in eliciting values for priority setting.

Bull (1991, p.38) argues that prioritisation or selection for treatment on the basis of QALY maximisation conflicts with our 'duty to care for all who suffer from ill health'. To put it in another way, Hadorn (1992, p.1454) suggests that the utilitarian 'greatest good for the greatest number' faces obstacles when it meets the 'rule of rescue', which he defines as 'the strong human proclivity to provide aid to identified victims of illness or accident'.

This problem of the interests of the individual versus the interests of the community is approached from two somewhat different directions. Drawing on theories of justice, ethicists are concerned that allocating resources to maximise aggregate health gain can over-ride the interests and rights of the individual (Doyal, 1995; Harris, 1987). Indeed, in a rather macabre example, Menzel (1990, p.15) points out that the sacrifice of an individual 'to extract vital organs and save four or five other people by transplant' would 'raise average life expectancy', i.e. increase health gain.

From the other more empirical direction, it is observed that the public are more sympathetic to a named individual in trouble than to unknown statistical individuals or, put another way, 'a named person who is dying now is more visible than an unnamed person dying in the future' (Welch and Larson, 1988, p.173). Indeed, although counter-instances can be identified, there are numerous examples where decisions have been made that place higher valuations on identified lives in immediate danger than on unknown lives in future danger – the 'statistical lives paradox' (Weale, 1979, p.186).

Fleck (1992, p.1608) describes, as an example of the inconsistent way in which society makes decisions, a mine where there are safety cuts to save money and thus preserve jobs, although it is known that these cuts place the lives of the miners at greater risk. However, despite the objective of saving money, in the event of a mine accident 'virtually no expense [is spared] in a rescue effort which we may well know is likely to be futile'. The analogy could be extended. Even had enormous resources been invested in mine safety, possibly because research had shown it to save far more lives per pound than rescue attempts, it is impossible to imagine a situation in which there would not be a major, no expense spared rescue attempt if subsequently, despite the safety expenditure, there were a disaster.

Some argue that 'society' must overcome its instincts – its sympathy for the named individual – and proceed with setting priorities to maximise health gain. Welch and Larson (1988, p.173) argue that the 'unidentified future patients need strong advocates in the medical community'. Others, however, acknowledge the existence of the 'duty to care' or the 'rule of rescue' and argue that it must be accommodated in any decisions about the allocation of healthcare resources.

This is a very difficult problem. It is quite correctly pointed out that, where resources are limited, expending a large amount of resources on one identified individual can deny those resources to others who might have achieved considerably more 'health gain' with them. Further, after extensive discussion of many aspects of this question, Weale (1979) concludes that the 'statistical lives paradox' does not constitute an ethical barrier to the principle of maximum benefit. However, can (or should) 'the strong human proclivity to provide aid to identified victims of illness or accident' be over-ridden? If 'society' persists with the 'rule of rescue', is 'society' wrong?

Attempts to explain the 'rule of rescue' or the 'statistical lives paradox' are often couched in terms of the greater emotional attachment to an identified individual rather than to as yet unidentified individuals, or sympathy for the individual in greater need as against a larger number in lesser need. Perhaps, however, certainty and risk play a part. Although not without controversy, mass vaccination can be advocated even where a small number of individuals will be severely damaged by the vaccine. The very low risk of severe injury is considered to be outweighed by the much higher risk of the disease against which the vaccination is given, resulting in a net health gain. But let us change the scenario slightly, if somewhat implausibly. Let us assume that it is known in advance which specific individuals are going to suffer severe damage but also that the only method of administering that vaccine requires that everyone is vaccinated, i.e. it is impossible to exclude any individual. All other factors (i.e. the severity of damage and number affected, the risk and severity of the disease being vaccinated against) remain the same, so the same net health gain would be achieved as in the earlier scenario. Would that mass vaccination programme still be advocated? If not, would this be solely because those who were to suffer severe injury were identified in advance? Or would the decision be affected by the related, but not identical, fact that what, in the original scenario, was a very low risk of severe injury for everyone is now a 100% certainty for a few and a zero risk for the many?

The conflict between the 'rule of rescue' and the maximisation of health gain was starkly illustrated in the debate surrounding the case of Jaymee Bowen, originally known only as Child B. The facts of this case are in dispute and it is claimed that the public debate was ill informed as to the actual details, although later comment (Price, 1996), informed by the All England Law Report, does not really support the ill-informed public argument. However, the important point for our discussion here lies in the terms of the public debate.

The Child B case, which remained headline news for several days in March 1995, came to prominence because the Cambridge Health Authority refused to pay for chemotherapy and a second bone marrow transplant (estimated to cost £75 000) for ten-year-old Jaymee Bowen, suffering from leukaemia. It was claimed by the

Cambridge and Huntingdon Health Commission* that this refusal was based on medical advice that the probability of success was extremely low (variously estimated at between 1% and 20%) and that 'this aggressive treatment would be detrimental to her quality of life' (Victor *et al.*, 1995). The alternative, Nigel Pitt (counsel for the health authority) is reported to have stated, 'was to adopt a palliative approach, enabling B to enjoy a few weeks or months of normal life' (Weale, 1995b). Had the reports gone no further than the first claim, i.e. that the refusal to pay for treatment was on purely medical grounds (especially if it had been argued that treatment would have been denied even if it were very cheap or even if there were no resource limitation), there would have been considerable public sympathy for the plight of the unfortunate victim, but the debate would probably have gone no further.**

The apparent precipitating factor for the ensuing debate came when the issue of limited resources and competing claims was raised explicitly. The Director of Health Policy and Public Health for the Cambridge and Huntingdon Health Commission is reported to have written: 'I considered that the substantial expenditure on treatment with such small prospect of success would not be effective use of resources. The amounts available for health care are not limitless' (Mullin, 1995), with the authority reportedly arguing that 'their cash reserves could better be spent on other patients' (Duce, 1995). This very firmly planted in people's minds the idea that the decision had been made on resource and not on medical grounds.

The ensuing debate in the press was a clear demonstration of the conflict between the 'rule of rescue' and the maximisation of health gain. While numerous contributors, both lay and medical, dwelt on the plight of the individual, health planners and public health doctors expounded the principles of rational resource allocation to maximise health gain within constrained resources.

It is no part of the discussion here to attempt to judge whether the original decision was made on resource or on medical grounds. However, the ensuing public debate did suggest a strong feeling that many members of society would not wish patients such as Jaymee Bowen to be denied (even heroic) treatment on the grounds of cost. Unless it can be argued that our society is too poor to treat cases such as Jaymee's, if the NHS is to take account of public opinion, it would appear that planners and purchasers need to balance the 'rule of rescue' against maximising health gain when allocating resources. The contrary argument, that the public must be informed and educated so that they will come to a rational opinion, may prove difficult to sustain. The public might not be wrong.[†]

---

* The Cambridge and Huntingdon Health Commission commissioned health services on behalf of the Cambridge and Huntingdon Health Authorities and the Cambridgeshire Family Health Services Authority.

** However, it was noted that the existence of the new language of the market-oriented health service might tend to make people less inclined to believe that decisions were purely medical (Victor and Penman, 1995).

[†] Jaymee Bowen's treatment was, in the event, paid for by an anonymous donor. Seven months later, with her leukaemia in remission and back at school, Jaymee was reported to have said: 'I'd rather have gone through more suffering to live than not go through anything and die' (Boseley, 1995). She had a further relapse and died in May 1996.

Earlier it was suggested that the 'rule of rescue' might be partly explained by moving from low risks for all to high (even 100%) risks for the identified individual. There is another area where risk and probability may play a part in the individual versus collective equation. Probabilities are quite properly applied to populations to calculate the potential health loss through a particular disease. Thus, for instance, a disease with a 1% probability of occurrence in any year, which reduced quality of life from 1 to 0.8 for one year, would be estimated to produce a health loss of 200 QALYs per year in a population of 100 000. Intervention costing a total £1 million per year to prevent or cure this disease would thus produce a corresponding health gain of 200 QALYs at a cost of £5000 per QALY. However, can probabilities be used in the same way in respect of an identified individual who, for example, has a 10% chance of of surviving for 20 years in perfect health (quality of life of 1) with treatment costing £100 000 but who without treatment will die immediately? Applying the same calculation as above, this treatment results in a cost per QALY of £50 000. Can this be compared with the cost per QALY of £5000 produced above? For the individual there is a 100% probability of dying without treatment. But the equation might get more complicated if the probability of cure were 1% or 0.1%.

Consideration of the 'rule of rescue' also leads us into ethical arguments surrounding 'letting die' through omission (withholding treatment) versus 'causing death' through commission. At present, even voluntary euthanasia is not permitted in most countries. However, should we not consider the possibility that acceptance of 'letting die' through failure to treat, even where the individual wishes that treatment and there is a finite probability of success, risks leading to compulsory euthanasia for those whose cost per QALY is deemed too high?

The dilemmas posed by this apparently insoluble problem are summarised by Callahan (1991, p.85) discussing the Oregon initiative:

> *The greatest source of anguish in the implementation of the plan will come in learning how to live with, and to rationalise, its failure to cover some people whose condition will pull at our sympathies. This anguish will be all the greater when the victims are visible and when the accountability for their condition cannot be evaded. This is the greatest logical and emotional problem created by any set of priorities that set limits.*

Outcomes not process

The health gain/QALY approach is criticised as being concerned solely with the outcomes of treatment and taking no account of benefits obtained from the process. For instance, it might seem reasonable to conclude that the benefit gained from IVF is a successful pregnancy. However, Ryan (1996a, p.549) found evidence of perceived benefit from going through treatment, even if the couple leaves childless. This objection can be accommodated by introducing the concept of 'process utility' or, as Dowie (1995) suggests, 'in-process outcome utility' and thus including such benefits in the 'health gain' achieved. Gerard and Mooney (1993) further suggest that QALYs fail to take account of non-health benefits including the receipt of information and reassurance.

Innovation

Concentration of resources on maximising health gain might jeopardize the introduction of new, potentially efficacious, treatments. For instance, in the early days, renal transplants would not have scored well on a QALY league table. To solve this problem there must be adequate provision, outside normal resource allocation, not only for research and development (R&D) but also for the transition from R&D to full 'production'.

Insurance

Potential patients, who have paid contributions to the healthcare system (under whatever contribution system prevails), may assume that they are purchasing 'assurance' that the healthcare will be provided when they need it. Whilst it is fashionable in some quarters to claim that we have a National Illness Service rather than a National Health Service and that this orientation should be changed, it may be that many people actually want, or expect, a National Illness Service. That is, they want, and consider they have paid for, a service which will 'pick them up and put them together' in case of catastrophe. Having paid their 'insurance' for such events, they may not be impressed by arguments that the process of 'picking them up and putting them together' scores too low on the cost-per-QALY scale. Rationing which leads to the denial of treatment could be considered to break the implicit contract.

This point was well expressed in a letter to the editor of *The Guardian* in connection with the Child B case. In that, the correspondent argued:

> *We are all contributing to an insurance scheme which we cannot rely on and which may let us down when we need it most . . . When we enter into an insurance contract for a house or a car, we expect the companies concerned to meet their obligations should the need arise and the premiums are set with this in mind. If the national health premiums are so low that the rationing of treatment has become unavoidable then this should be addressed rather than limiting treatment by arbitrary funding levels and cost effective criteria.* (Turley, 1995)

Should QALYs and health gain be abandoned?

Despite all the objections outlined above, QALYs and the concept of health gain are probably too valuable to be ignored. However, their dangers must be recognised. Despite the recognition, quoted above, that 'there will be a need for a purchasing authority to form a view about what weight it will attach to equity concerns relative to those of efficiency' (Mooney *et al.*, 1992, p.9), the appearance of scientific exactness of QALYs, combined with the power of numbers, creates the danger that the quantitative QALYs will prevail over the qualitative notions of equity, fairness and justice. This danger is foreshadowed in the later statement by Mooney *et al.* (1992, p.9) that 'There are no hard and fast rules with respect to equity. Unlike efficiency there are no precise guidelines for its pursuit'.

In contrast to the pursuit of efficiency and frequent unquestioning acceptance by many UK commentators of maximisation of health gain as an objective, the Swedish Parliamentary Priorities Commission (1995, p.21) considers that the principles of human dignity and of need and solidarity over-ride the cost-efficiency principle. Thus, they conclude that cost-efficiency principles 'cannot justify refraining from or impairing the quality of the care given to the dying, the severely and chronically ill, old persons, dementia patients, the mentally retarded, the severely handicapped or other persons for whom care would not "pay"'.

Maximising health gain is often presented as a technical or formulaic approach to priority setting, thus leaving little scope for public involvement. Public values are often involved in valuing the health states used in constructing QALYs and similar measures. However, public involvement which manifests itself as the 'rule of rescue' is seen by some to indicate that the public must be educated to suppress its sympathies and act rationally.

Rationing by exclusion

Explicit rationing is frequently associated with rationing by exclusion (i.e. identifying services and treatments which will not be supplied at all (at least to certain groups)). It is worth noting, however, that all healthcare systems have to determine their limits, i.e. what treatments they do and do not cover. These limits vary between countries, as does what does and does not constitute health and healthcare. For instance, some health systems in continental Europe include spa treatment, whilst such treatment is no longer provided within the NHS. Few would label its omission as rationing.

There have been several recent attempts to introduce or propose 'limited lists', 'defined packages', 'core services' within healthcare, each using different bases or criteria for inclusion or exclusion from the list or package.

Probably the best known is the Oregon plan.* The Oregon Basic Health Services Act, passed in 1989, aimed *inter alia* to provide Medicaid to all those with incomes below the Federal Poverty Level (FPL) instead of only to those with incomes below 58% of the FPL, the limit prevailing within the state at that time (Honigsbaum, 1991, pp.8–9). To

---

*There have been numerous accounts of the Oregon plan and so it will be mentioned here only briefly.

do this without substantially increasing total costs meant that rationing by excluding sections of the poor would be replaced by rationing by excluding some forms of treatment. To effect this, a Health Services Commission was created, charged with drawing up a 'list of health services ranked in priority ... according to the comparative benefits of each service to the entire population being served' (Kitzhaber, 1993, p.375). According to the funds available, a line was to be drawn on this list. Condition/treatment pairs above this line would be provided to all those eligible; those below the line would not be provided. The first attempt to produce a prioritised list employed a cost-utility (cost-effectiveness) approach (effectively a form of cost per QALY), informed by consultation with the public via a telephone survey, public hearings and community meetings. However, as noted earlier, this initial or draft list was widely criticised for, among other things, its apparently counter-intuitive rankings. The revised final priority list owed far more to the judgement of the commissioners and was generated without reference to costs (Hadorn, 1991b, p.2218). Having received the necessary Federal Waivers, the Oregon Plan was implemented on 1 February 1994 adding, according to its architect (Kitzhaber and Kemmy, 1995, p.817), 'over 115 000 newly eligible Oregonians to the ranks of those receiving care though Medicaid'.

The Dunning Committee (the Committee on Choices in Health Care) in the Netherlands was charged with examining ways of limiting new technologies, dealing with scarcity and rationing care. It proposed that treatments and services to be included in a basic package of healthcare should conform to four criteria – or pass through four sieves. The first sieve retains (i.e. excludes) unnecessary care, with the Committee arguing that 'the extent to which a type of care is necessary must be established by the community-oriented approach' (Dunning, 1992, p.84). Necessary care includes services which guarantee normal functioning as a member of the community, services which maintain or restore ability to participate in social activities, services to prevent serious injury to health in the long term. The second sieve retains (excludes) care with unconfirmed effectiveness or confirmed ineffectiveness; the third sieve selects (allows to pass) on efficiency, using cost-effectiveness and cost-utility analysis; the final sieve excludes 'care that may be left to individual responsibility and individual payment' (Dunning, 1992, pp.85–6; Scheerder, 1993, p.53).

As part of extensive 'reforms' to the New Zealand health services, a 'national health committee', which has gone under a range of official titles, was established charged with providing independent advice on priorities in publicly funded health services. Initially, this committee came under pressure to produce a relatively simple list of 'core services' which would be provided by the publicly funded health system (Hadorn and Holmes, 1997). However, the 'harsh reality' of many of the problems posed by the inclusion/exclusion list approach, outlined below, dampened the 'early enthusiasm for the advantages of a clear and explicit list' (Cooper, 1995, p.804). In the event, the committee recommended 'that "core" be defined as being what was already being provided prior to the reports and set about establishing what precisely that was'. The concept of a fixed list of core services to be publicly funded was abandoned to be replaced by a 'qualified list' setting out the clinical circumstances which are deemed appropriate for a given treatment (Cooper, 1995, p.805). According to Hadorn and Holmes (1997, p.132), eligibility for services is defined:

> in terms of clinical practice guidelines or explicit assessment criteria which depict the circumstances under which patients are likely to derive substantial health benefit from those services, bearing in mind competing claims on resources.

New and Le Grand (1996) argue in favour of defining a package of healthcare services that the NHS is responsible for. To determine what should be included in such a package, they turn to the characteristics of healthcare that make it special, different from other commodities and services. These characteristics they identify as unpredictability, information imbalance and fundamental importance. In order to be included in the package they argue that healthcare services must meet all three criteria. According to their analysis, fertility treatment, continuing medical care and curative dental treatment satisfy all three criteria and should be included; the provision of spectacles, hearing aids and medicines for non-complex conditions do not and thus should not be included. Defining such a package, they argue, says nothing about the effectiveness or value for money of the services included. 'It simply clarifies what the NHS should be in the business of doing' (New, 1997, p.505).

There have been attempts, most notably in Oregon, to obtain public views to inform the selection of criteria for the prioritisation or inclusion/exclusion of treatments. However, there have also been attempts to elicit public views directly on the relative priority to be given to particular treatments, rather than on the criteria to inform prioritisation (see, for instance, Bowling *et al.*, 1993; Heginbotham, 1993). These approaches raise serious questions about whether the public, or indeed anyone, can meaningfully answer such questions, about how such answers should be interpreted and about how views so elicited can or should be used in decision making. This latter point relates closely to the prior consent argument discussed in Chapter Three and below. One authority, at least, has been recommended by its Director of Public Health to 'back a local survey which concluded routine NHS funding of fertility treatment should cease'. The survey is reported to have shown that 'most people saw assisted conception services as the lowest priority' (Hall, 1997).

A defined package of services, a limited list or a clear cut-off point – rationing by exclusion – whilst appearing attractive by making eligibility for treatment explicit and transparent, raises a wide range of practical and ethical problems.

Marginal versus average

The heterogeneity of patients can cause problems where some forms of treatment, or some condition/treatment pairs, are completely excluded on the justification of maximising health gain. For instance, if QALY league tables are drawn up on the basis of average benefit per pound and priorities are determined by treating the conditions with the lowest average cost per QALY before proceeding to conditions with higher average cost per QALY, or by simply excluding the treatments with the highest cost per QALY, no allowance is made for variability in the severity of cases or in the capacity of individual patients to benefit. Thus whilst the excluded treatments may, on average, yield fewer QALYs per pound, this may not be true for individual cases at the margin. This could lead to a situation where one patient is treated to little beneficial effect simply because the treatment is included on the list or is 'above the cut-off line', whilst another patient is denied treatment from which they could receive considerable benefit simply because that treatment is excluded from the list or is 'below the cut-off line'.

Hyland and Crocker (1995) give the example of the drug salmeterol used in asthma treatment. Clinical trials show that the drug, although effective, is much more so for some patients than for others. However, there has been little research to determine which particular groups benefit most.

To avoid the 'averaging' problem, Gerard and Mooney (1993, p.62) state that:

> Underlying the use of [QALY] league tables in health care policy making is the idea that each possible health care programme should ideally be provided at a level at which the ratio of marginal costs to QALYs is the same across all activities.

However, in addition to questioning what QALYs actually measure, they report that lack of evidence makes it difficult to judge the adequacy of the marginal analysis in many of the CUA (cost-utility analysis) studies used to compile league tables.

Accuracy of diagnosis

Any justification for the total exclusion of some treatment/condition pairs must be predicated on accurate diagnosis. However, if the exclusion encompasses the initial referral to a specialist, it is possible that serious conditions might be missed where the original diagnosis is faulty. Concern over a case of 'rationing by lifestyle' was heightened by the fact that the patient, a heavy smoker, was denied not only treatment but the diagnostic tests which would have revealed the seriousness of his condition (Ward, 1993). In a hypothetical example, if specialist treatment for lower back pain was excluded from the list of permitted treatments, a GP faced with a patient presenting with that complaint, but who does not suspect the underlying cause of cancer, might feel it not worth referring that patient to a specialist. In this context, it is interesting to note that Oregon will provide 'initial evaluation and diagnosis for all conditions' (Kitzhaber, 1993, p.377). However, 'creep' in medical diagnosis, whether intentional or unintentional, could sabotage rationing by exclusion by ensuring that the diagnosis and treatment fell within the 'included' list.

Co-morbidities

Rationing by exclusion, taken to its logical conclusion, could lead to absurdities where a person is suffering simultaneously from one condition for which treatment is excluded and one for which treatment is included. They could die of one condition whilst being treated for the other.

Ability to pay

Possibly more than any other method, rationing by exclusion effectively means rationing by ability to pay, which was discussed in Chapter Two. For example, using the much-maligned waiting lists as a rationing mechanism does at least mean that patients with low-priority conditions have a choice between waiting and paying. If low-priority, or indeed any other, conditions are excluded completely, the only choice is between no treatment and paying.

Van De Ven (1995, p.788), however, considers that a two-tier health system, in which those who can pay receive excluded treatments whilst those who cannot pay do not receive those treatments, whilst arguably threatening solidarity and equity, is inevitable. 'Those who can pay will always find their way, abroad or in their own country.' Given this, he prefers a system in which everyone has immediate access to specified services rather than a system apparently providing all services but with long waiting lists for some of them.

Priority setting by age

It is claimed that some approaches to rationing, in particular maximising health gain, constitute (systematic) discrimination against certain groups – the poor, the old, ethnic minorities, one gender or the other, those living in remote areas. However, it would be very difficult to find anyone who advocated, as a matter of principle, discriminating against the poor, an ethnic minority group or women, although there are occasional arguments that those living in remote areas choose to do so, gain benefits from doing so and thus cannot also expect equal services.

In contrast, rationing by age appears to be viewed in a different light, sometimes by arguing that rationing by age does not constitute discrimination since everyone will be (or has a finite probability of being) old, unlike being a woman or a member of an ethnic minority. Further, the high costs of caring for growing numbers of older people can 'produce strong incentives for rationing publicly funded health care based on age' (Jecker, 1991, p.3012).

Some commentators have argued that the NHS has an inbuilt tendency to discriminate against older people. One of the most frequently cited examples is treatment for endstage renal failure (ESRF). Baker (1993, p.143) presents data to show that age-specific acceptance rates for ESRF in the UK were lower at all ages than in other countries but very much lower for the over-64 group. Indeed, in all other countries the rate goes up with age but in the UK it drops above age 64. Baker asks if age rationing is unfair in principle.

A rather extreme argument is attributed to Governor Richard Lamm of Colorado, who is quoted as stating in 1984 that elderly people 'have a duty to die and get out of the way. Let the other society, our kids, build a reasonable life' (Arcangelo, 1994, p.26). Whilst few would be so blunt, it is suggested that age discrimination could be justified on the basis of the fair innings argument. As described by Harris (1988, p.119), 'This argument concentrates on the idea that it cannot be just that someone who has already had more than his or her fair share of life and its delights should be preferred to the younger person who has not been so favoured'. Indeed, Lockwood (1988), who favours the fair innings argument, suggests that QALYs are not sufficiently ageist as they do not take this argument into account. The fair innings argument is based on the view that some span of years constitutes a reasonable life and that anyone who does not reach that age suffers the injustice of missing out on a reasonable share of life. Anyone reaching that threshold has received their entitlement – 'The rest of their life is a sort of bonus which may be cancelled when this is necessary to help others reach the threshold' (Harris, 1985, p.91). However, Harris goes on to suggest that the fairness underlying this argument can become 'a reason for always preferring to save younger rather than older people, whatever the age difference' (p.92).

Callahan (1993) suggests setting an age limit on the most expensive high-technology procedures, whilst improving long-term and home care. Denial of care, he argues, does not constitute disrespect for the elderly as death is tolerable once a 'natural lifespan' has been lived (Callahan, 1987, p.172).

Williams (1997) applies the fair innings argument to life expectancy but further argues that it should embrace quality-adjusted life expectancy (QALE). Thus, to achieve a fair innings – to equalise QALEs – groups with a lower health status throughout life would need to live longer to achieve their fair innings than groups with a higher health status.

In almost direct contrast to the fair innings argument is the argument of just rewards – that age discrimination is not just because of the past contributions made to society or, more specifically, to the NHS by the elderly (Harrison and Hunter, 1994).

Rather more pragmatic are the economic arguments in favour of discriminating against the elderly. Younger people, it is argued, 'are relatively more productive and efficient in their contributions to society', more life-years are gained from treating younger people and, since the elderly, on average, consume more healthcare resources, greater savings are made from denying care to the old (Jecker and Pearlman, 1989, p.1070). Against this, however, Jecker and Pearlman argue that 'We value persons not merely as means to productive or efficient output, but as ends-in-themselves'. Further, they argue that 'even if the social worth of persons is simply a function of their productive contribution, many older people could be far more productive than they are now if social barriers were removed'.

A further pragmatic argument for age discrimination suggests that, as elderly people are less able to benefit from treatment, less health gain will be achieved. Against this, Evans (1991) claims that there is a persistent misunderstanding of the link between age and ability to benefit from high-technology medicine. Although on average older patients do less well after hazardous medical or surgical interventions, this does not affect everyone equally and thus should not be used as a basis for discrimination. He argues that physiological status is the main predictor of outcome and that age adds very little. Thus patients should be assessed for treatment on the basis of their physiology and not their chronological age.

Public views on rationing by age have often been elicited by inviting respondents to choose between two people of different ages when treatment is available for only one of them. Posing such questions in terms of individuals, in any case, risks being influenced by the 'rule of rescue' effect and is thus unlikely to offer much valid information on the general issue of age discrimination. Evans (1997, p.823), whilst noting that surveys in Britain suggest that older people are viewed as having lower social worth than younger people, totally rejects any suggestion that these public attitudes constitute a valid basis for rationing in the NHS.

Rationing by prior consent

Chapter Two examined the argument that rationing can be just and fair provided that there is prior consent. It was questioned whether, within the NHS, it would be possible to create a situation in which users could be deemed to have freely given their prior consent to restrictions. There are, however, further problems raised by the prior consent approach.

Fleck (1994b, p.380) states that a requirement for rational democratic deliberation as an approach to healthcare rationing is that 'We must be largely ignorant of our future health care needs, which is largely true for most of us most of the time'. He further (1992, pp.1632–3) argues that 'the vast majority of us are like Rawl's disembodied spirits behind the veil of ignorance. We are capable of a rare degree of impartiality because we really do not know enough about our future health needs'.

However, Menzel (1992, p.22) argues that there are problems with congenital or early-onset conditions as decision makers would be 'dealing with a condition they knew they would not one day have. That is, they would not be making their rationing choices in a fair, risk-taking state of ignorance about how the resulting allocations will turn out individually for them in particular'. Further, there is a gender dimension as men know they will not get diseases specific to women and vice versa. With current genetic research increasing our potential knowledge about predisposition to illness, the 'veil of ignorance' argument may become increasingly hard to sustain. This raises problems about the free choice of health plan. Those with pre-existing disability or with a known predisposition to illness will select health plans with few restrictions, whilst the more healthy will be happy to accept restrictions in return for lower premiums. The cost and equity implications are obvious.

Even if all problems about group decision making can be overcome, how far can the argument that prior consent to rationing will make it not only just but acceptable be maintained in practice, especially in the face of the 'rule of rescue'? Fleck (1992, p.1624) argues that:

> if our rationing protocols are the products of an informed democratic consensus, then any such alleged 'duty to rescue' is morally specious at best and morally pernicious at worst because a just consensus about healthcare rationing will be violated.

However, let us return to the mine safety analogy, discussed above. Even if the miners themselves (individually or collectively) had freely agreed in advance to the spending of safety money on the understanding there would be no money left for rescue attempts, it is unthinkable that, on the grounds of cost, there would be no attempt to rescue trapped miners in the event of a disaster.

The above arguments are made mostly within the US context. However, in the light of the current UK debates about rationing, it is interesting to note that several US commentators (for instance, Daniels (1991)) have remarked on the apparent consensus and acceptance within the (pre-1991) NHS of the (implicit) rationing involved. Indeed, Aaron and Schwartz (1990, p.422) argue:

> the British experience with rationing, particularly stark because of its severity, sharply delineates the kinds of choices we shall have to make. Understanding how the British make these decisions can help us find ways to make our less extreme but still painful choices acceptable.

On the other hand, Crawshaw (1990, p.663) characterises rationing within the NHS as 'a dense, obscurating bureaucracy, intentionally avoiding written policy for macroallocation (rationing), and a publicly unaccountable medical profession privately managing microallocation so as to conceal life and death decisions from patients'.

Prioritising waiting lists

There has recently been considerable interest in prioritising waiting lists, to determine both the order of selection from the list and eligibility to join the list. A method for prioritising waiting lists in Salisbury, which has aroused considerable interest, sums the squares of the scores that patients receive in each of five categories: speed of disease; pain or distress; disability or dependence on others; loss of occupation; and time waiting (Edwards, 1994). Gudex et al. (1990) proposed a method of prioritising waiting lists according to QALY gain and resource use. Elwyn et al. (1996) report an assessment of the clinical priority of patients on an orthopaedic waiting list based on judgements of pain and disability. Labour, when in opposition, was reported to have proposed prioritising waiting lists, on the analogy of waiting lists for housing, with clinical needs graded on a ten-point scale (Dobson, 1993).

There is nothing new in this idea. A number of waiting list prioritisation formulae were proposed in the late 1960s and early 1970s. These included a formula devised by the Institute for Operational Research (IOR) (Luckman *et al.*, 1969) which took the form:

$$P = S^a \, D \, T_w^{\,b}$$

which was later simplified by Phoenix (1972, p.80) to:

$$P = D \, T^{\sqrt{w}}$$

> where   S = social factor
>   D = disability factor
>   W = deterioration factor
>   T = time on waiting list
>   a & b are constants

Another formula, used by the Birmingham RHB OR Unit (Eltringham and Clare, 1973), took the form:

$$P = 800(1 - e^{-kT})$$

> where   k = f (urgency)
>   T = time on waiting list

This latter formula was implemented at a district general hospital to select patients from the waiting list according to their priority score, taking into account theatre and bed scheduling requirements. However, the lack of availability of local computing facilities at that time militated against long-term survival of the system.

However, some of the relatively simple systems such the Salisbury approach carry with them the danger that their apparent precision will mislead people into giving them far more credit than is due – they may become elevated to scientific truths – and their underlying logic and legitimacy may receive too little attention.

Involving the public in priority setting: the legitimate scope for local priorities

At the national level the public should be able to influence decisions on total health-care (or at least NHS) expenditure and the overall philosophy and scope of the health service through the democratic political process, possibly supplemented by other forms of participation which are national in scope.

However, spurred on by *Local Voices* (DoH, 1992), most interest in involving the public in healthcare priority setting in the UK has been at the local level, mainly health authority but sometimes at trust and GP practice level. This, however, leads us into the debate about whether, within a national health service, healthcare priorities should be determined at the local level. In recent years emphasis from the DoH has been that priorities should be determined locally, a line Maynard (1996a) terms irresponsible. Under the slogan of 'Meeting local needs', health authorities had been encouraged to engage with their public locally and, individually, to determine local priorities and to select locally what to purchase. Whilst the 1997 White Paper *The New NHS* (DoH, 1997) promises a 'genuinely *national* service' with National Services Frameworks so that 'patients will get greater consistency in the availability and quality of services, right across the NHS' (para 7.8), the securing of services will remain a local responsibility, within the framework of local Health Improvement Programmes. Where the resulting balance between national and local priorities will fall will not become apparent for some time.

Emphasis on local priorities has been criticised as it may permit the centre (the government) to shift the blame for the lack of provision of a specific service or even for a general shortage of resources. As Pollock (1995, p.475) expresses it: 'Priority setting exercises seek to legitimise cost containment by asking local communities to identify those services they would be most prepared to forgo'.

Another major concern arises because of the threat to inter-district equity. Unless priorities are based solely on some nationally agreed definition of need applied to local population needs, determining priorities locally will lead to differences between health authorities in what services they choose to secure and, more importantly, choose not to secure. This results in unequal access to services dependent only on place of residence. It can be questioned whether the concept of locally determined priorities is compatible with a national health service. A corollary of locally determined differential purchasing priorities is that doctors find their 'duty' to treat according to clinical priority compromised.

At the same time it has to be recognised that, even within a national health service, equity would not be achieved by having identical services in every area. There are many legitimate reasons why different services are needed to meet the different needs of local populations and thus ensure geographical equity. Box 4.2 suggests legitimate and non-legitimate 'justifications' for variations in services between health districts. Within the suggested list of legitimate justifications for variations, apart from the more technical aspects relating to demography and epidemiology, most aspects relate to the way in which services are delivered, rather than which services are delivered. However, Box 4.2 suggests it is open to question whether, within a national health service, it is legitimate for local views or values to result in inter-district or inter-locality variations in the services provided.

Many legitimate justifications relate to 'objective' demographic differences which affect 'need', such as the size, composition and morbidity of the local population. Such differences clearly require local variations in service provision in order to achieve inter-district (or inter-primary care group) equity – to ensure that people living in different locations, but in otherwise identical circumstances with identical health needs, are not treated differently. However, it is not self-evidently clear that there is a role here for public or consumer participation, beyond any role in determining morbidity levels and drawing attention to unidentified needs.

Box 4.2: Some justifications for variations in services between districts within a National Health Service

Legitimate justification
- Size and demographic characteristics of population
- Epidemiology/disease patterns
- Ethnic/religious differences
- Level of car ownership
- Population density and natural barriers
- Public transport
- Level of economic activity, especially of women
- Climate
- Socioeconomic factors
- Quality of housing
- Provision and quality of other services

Non-legitimate justification
- Historical patterns of provision and/or usage
- Values/choices/views of local health authority/commission

Justifications whose legitimacy is open to question
- Values/views of local population
- Level of private health insurance
- Values and/or views of local GPs

Other justifications for variations relate to process factors in the way that services are delivered, which may affect access to services and the acceptability of those services to users. Here there would appear to be a clear role for public and consumer participation. However, even in this relatively unproblematic area of priority setting in the way that services are provided, questions of the 'dictatorship of the majority' could arise if, for instance, majority preference for a particular mode of delivery was used to justify imposing that model of delivery on everyone. Further, it should be recognised that there is a distinction between collective participation in influencing the general pattern of the way that services are provided and individual 'participation' to ensure services received are acceptable to them as an individual. At this individual level the major role for participation is empowerment of patients to allow them to take more control over their treatment, including making informed choices between alternatives.

What is far more questionable, however, is how far local views or values should be permitted to lead to variations in which services are provided, which are not justified by the demographic factors identified above.

Let us illustrate this more concretely with strictly hypothetical examples. Should the fact that a sample (however carefully drawn) of the public in Buckingham values hip replacements higher than CABGs, whilst a similar sample of the public in Norfolk rates CABGs above hip replacements, lead to the policy conclusion that Buckingham should purchase relatively fewer CABGs and Norfolk should purchase relatively fewer hip replacements?* Similarly, would the fact that a sample of the public in Cambridge responds that *mutatis mutandis*, treatment of a young person should take precedence over treatment of an old person, whilst Oxford respondents give higher priority to the old person, justify the local health authorities in purchasing to favour the young and the old, respectively? Should the fact that a sample of Mayerbridge residents feels that AIDS sufferers should receive no treatment or care affect the local health authority's purchasing pattern? Or a slightly more realistic example – should treatment for smokers receive lower priority in those locations where public consultation has suggested such lower priority?

Indeed, Evans (1993, p.50) goes further and argues that an approach that puts the rights of individual citizens in the hands of other citizens is fallacious. He continues:

> *The rights of an individual should be embodied in the constitution of the state . . . One of the principles of the British state is that all citizens are equal in having equal status before the law and equal basic access to the means of life, education and health . . . Such rights should not be withdrawn from the citizens of this country by any means other than formal Act of Parliament.*

Scope for public and consumer participation in priority setting

If we return to Box 4.1, which listed areas of priority setting within the NHS, we see that some form of consumer or public participation is indicated, to a lesser or greater extent, in all of them. However, for many areas the appropriate form of participation is at the national level via the normal democratic political process supplemented, as appropriate, by national forms of public participation. In other areas the appropriate form of participation would appear to be individual patient empowerment. Between these lie areas where the legitimacy of public and consumer participation, especially insofar as it relates to local variations in which services are provided, is still open to debate.

---

* Of course, it is a different issue where the respondents give hip replacements, CABGs or any other treatment a high priority because their locality is currently undersupplied relative to the rest of the UK, taking into account local morbidity. The example here assumes the respondents value hip replacements more highly than CABGs *per se* (or vice versa), independently of the local supply situation.

CHAPTER FIVE

Engaging the public

Recent trends in public involvement

Issues of consumer involvement in healthcare and the question of whether it is appropriate, or indeed a right, for the public to be involved in decisions about health policy were discussed in Chapters Three and Four. However, these issues have become more sharply focused in recent years as priority setting has emerged as a key element in health systems.

Traditionally within the NHS, doctors holding an elite and respected position in society made decisions on behalf of their patients on the grounds that they alone had the specialist knowledge to do so and because they were assumed to act in the best interests of the patient.

Over the years, a whole range of special interest or user groups has emerged. Such groups are often highly knowledgeable and, at times, successful in influencing the nature of services. However, because they are often motivated by personal experience their influence may be constrained by being seen as obviously self-interested and thereby unrepresentative.

The relationship between doctor, patient and the wider community, and the legitimacy with which they view each other's roles, are strongly influenced by the historical context of the development of the medical profession. This historical context serves to shape the attitudes of different groups both to public participation in health policy decisions and to how much involvement should be undertaken. However, in addition to influences specific to health services, general forces for change in public service accountability (a more educated population and growing consumerism) have been credited with increasing interest in public involvement.

In 1992 the government published *Local Voices*, a White Paper describing the need to involve the public in purchasing decisions (DoH, 1992). Whilst this represented an explicit statement about priority setting, it was not quite as explicit in practice as the subsequent debate became. The following abstract illustrates this point.

If Health Authorities are to establish a champion of the people role, their decisions should reflect, so far as practical, what people want, their preferences, concerns and values. Being responsive to local views will enhance the credibility of health authorities but, more importantly, is likely to result in services which are better suited to local needs and therefore more appropriate. There may of course be occasions when local views have to be over-ridden (eg on the weight of epidemiological, resource or other considerations) and in such circumstances, it is important that Health Authorities explain the reasons for their decisions.

Moreover, as Health Authorities seek to bring about changes in services and make explicit decisions about priorities they are likely to be more persuasive and successful in their negotiations with providers if they secure public support. (DoH, 1992, p.3)

There is in this policy statement considerable emphasis on providing information to local people, on learning what the public value in terms of healthcare and on utilising community knowledge as a basis for explaining decisions. It was not at this stage very explicit about the public engaging in explicit rationing or, indeed, about how the public view was to be captured.

However, the strands of change in the health system were inevitably beginning to interact to produce a more insistent requirement to engage the public in establishing healthcare priorities. Health authorities found themselves under increasing financial pressure and were being asked to set priorities in terms of the clinical and cost-effectiveness of particular services. As discussed in Chapter Four, there was growing interest in the work undertaken in Oregon. In addition, early attempts to restrict treatment for non-life threatening conditions, such as removal of tattoos, varicose vein surgery and fertility treatment, had aroused considerable publicity. Cambridge and Huntingdon Health Commission's decision not to fund further treatment for Child B and the subsequent appeal resulted in the the High Court Judge commenting that 'Responsible Authorities must do more than toll the bell of tight resources – they must explain the priorities that have led them to decline to fund treatment' (Roberts *et al.*, 1996).

Around the same time the Royal College of Physicians issued a report which stated that 'It is a requirement of a democratic society that the public, as well as the professions and the politicians, should be involved in any debate over priorities in health care' (RCP, 1995, p.11).

There was then growing advocacy that the public should be involved in specific priority-setting decisions, as summarised by the set of arguments listed in Box 5.1.

The basic thrust of such arguments is that of enhancing legitimacy for priority-setting decisions. These arguments exist at two levels. The first and more abstract level, which was addressed in Chapter Three, is that of the democratic principle and, at least theoretically, applies to all decisions in a democratic society. The second level assumes that meaningful and reliable data can be gathered about specific decisions. This leads directly to the questions of who are the public and how they can be involved in the decisions.

Box 5.1:   Prioritising services: arguments for involving the public

- As a publicly funded service, the NHS should be answerable to its actual and potential consumers (Donovan and Coast, 1994).
- In order to fulfil their role as 'champion of the people', health authorities must demonstrate that they are capable of consulting widely and tackling difficult resource allocation decisions in a public arena (Heginbotham *et al.*, 1993).
- The public may have different perceptions of issues from clinicians and it is essential that the public voice is heard to avoid a unitary and potentially biased professional view (Heginbotham *et al.*, 1993).
- Appropriate and effective services are more likely to be developed if framed on the basis of needs identified in conjunction with users (NHSE *et al.*, 1998).
- Greater public involvement in resource allocation decisions may lead to a widening consensus about priorities (NHSE *et al.*, 1998).
- As the information relating to clinical effectiveness and outcomes grows, there is a need both to inform patients and to ensure that the information itself reflects the patients' perspective on the benefits of their treatment (NHSE, 1996b).

Who should be involved and how?

As discussed in Chapter Four, priority setting arises in many different areas of the NHS (see Box 4.1). Before embarking on any exercise to involve the public in priority setting, it is essential to be very clear about its purpose: the area of priority setting, the decisions to be made and how the 'results' of public involvement might influence the decision making. The purpose of the exercise will, in turn, determine the choice of method and which section of the 'public' should be involved – the 'target population'. For some purposes, citizen involvement will be indicated; for others, collective user or even individual patient views will be required.

The influence of the purpose and area of application on the choice of both method and who should be involved is illustrated in a joint publication by the NHSE, the Institute of Health Services Management and the NHS Confederation (1998), which attempts to describe a strategy for public involvement. It outlines four general models.

- *Direct participation by users* – where great emphasis and potential value are given to an improved collaboration between health providers, particularly clinicians, and patients in their own treatment regime.
- *Informed views of citizens* – which outlines approaches to improving the knowledge base of the public and then subsequently engaging them in debate about health and health services.
- *Community development* – which is a wide and holistic construct where local

communities are encouraged to participate in and influence their health status but not solely through health service activities.

- *Local scrutiny and accountability* – which attempts to establish a sense of responsibility for the patient's experience of health services at a local level rather than from a national perspective.

However, whilst there is much of value here in addressing the basic democratic deficit surrounding healthcare, there is a sense that the models above do not get to grips with the really difficult aspects of priority setting. Even the second model, which is perhaps the most relevant approach in the current context, is advocated at the general level of enhanced dialogue, enhanced commitment and ownership and improved capacity for informed debate. Indeed, a word of caution is offered by the authors, who suggest that:

> *The model is unlikely to be the most useful approach . . . for taking decisions as opposed to contributing to the decision-making process – the model should not be seen as a way of abrogating statutory responsibilities for decision-making.* (p.14)

Taking a slightly different approach, public involvement can be thought of as existing along a broad spectrum, as indicated in Box 5.2. At one end, individual patients can engage in personal decisions about their own treatment pattern and ultimately perhaps improve the overall pattern of particular services. In this latter capacity, they may be best thought of as acting in an extended or proxy consumer role. Towards the opposite end of the spectrum there is the citizen role, operating in a more collective way to influence and determine services which may or may not be made available to their fellow citizens. This form of 'hard choices' priority setting or rationing is the focus of this text but it is as well to recognise that this is part of a spectrum and in practice areas can overlap.

Box 5.2:   Levels of public involvement in the NHS

- Ethos/values of health system
  (rights v rewards)
  (total expenditure on health)

- What healthcare services/treatments should be provided
  (what is, and is not, included within the health service)

- How and where health services are to be provided
  (locally v regionally)
  (institution v community)

- Non-medical aspects
  (appointment systems, waiting, food, decor)

- Individual choice of treatment
  (individual involvement, empowerment)

The importance of ensuring the identification of the 'target population' appropriate to the purposes of the project is further emphasised by Lomas (1997). He argues (p.5) that whichever group is used is likely 'to make a difference to the type of answer one receives'. Studies indicate that the general public is less likely to prioritise healthcare to conditions where the individual may be perceived to have contributed, e.g. drug addiction, lung cancer (Richardson *et al.*, 1992). Another study by Hopton and Dlugolecka (1995) reports that, whereas patients gave second ranked priority to 'help or advice about pain management', this was placed 12th by the general public. Many other incongruencies might be identified. Such a finding is not really surprising since individuals with different backgrounds may have quite different views. Moreover, these views may well change over time as they have different experiences.

In some cases, even when the purpose of the exercise has been defined fairly clearly, it will not be immediately apparent which is the most appropriate target population. As mentioned in Chapter Four, this arises particularly when valuing health states; should the values be those of the general public, who may or may not have had experience of those health states, or should values be restricted to those of people with current or past experience of the states? Although careful consideration of the objectives of the exercise will help in determining which is the most appropriate target population, controversy is likely to remain.

Notwithstanding the fundamental importance of ensuring that the appropriate 'target population' is identified, the focus of attention of most of the literature has shifted to the question of how information should be collected; are some methods better than others in producing reliable and valid data and does the choice of method actually influence the outcome obtained? Before looking at methods, it is worth restating that we are concerned here with the public role in determining which services should be provided and to whom. We are not in this instance primarily concerned with issues such as patient satisfaction where to some extent the focus of the information required is more clearly defined. However, many methodologies discussed here are also applicable to this latter area.

The fundamental issue when selecting particular methods is again the intention or purpose of the involvement. The views of informed service users about a particular treatment may well be gathered in a very different way from an attempt to obtain views about setting priorities for services available to a local community. The interaction between the purpose of the involvement and the method chosen is likely to influence the overall perceived legitimacy of the process. We will return to this point in the final chapter.

Specific methods and their value in priority setting

Following the 1991 changes in the NHS, the main responsibility to ensure public involvement fell, as a result of government initiatives, to health authorities in their dual task of trying to assess health need and then delivering the most relevant services within available resources. This situation led to a substantial amount of activity, characterised by a great diversity of approach which has raised major issues of both method and cost (Lupton *et al.*, 1998, p.100). Perhaps, however, this diversity and subsequent mismatch between the views of the public and the professionals has been used as an excuse to avoid or undervalue public involvement (Flynn *et al.*, 1996).

Chapter Seven provides an account of findings from research aimed at establishing what health authorities in the UK have done in involving the public in healthcare priority setting and what has been achieved by this process. The rest of this chapter will discuss some methods of engaging the public and Chapter Six will explore methods of eliciting values in more depth.

A very wide range of approaches can be, and have been, used for 'involving' the public in the NHS and some of these are listed in Box 5.3. However, broadly, the nature of methods for engaging the public is parallel to the whole domain of social enquiry and the methods used are those of the social scientist, detailed accounts of which (for example, Frankfort-Nachmias and Nachmias, 1996; Parahoo, 1997) should be consulted prior to undertaking an active investigation. The purpose here is simply to identify the main approaches, illustrate potential usage and comment upon their suitability as techniques for engaging the public.

Quantitative versus qualitative methods

Quantitative approaches are frequently posed against qualitative approaches although several methodologies straddle the divide. Given the orientation of priority setting, or the notion of choosing between one activity and another, there is a sense that obtaining quantitative data would be valuable in clarifying the weighting or strength of feeling about a particular option. We shall see that qualitative methods may be equally useful in particular contexts but the dominant quantitative method – the survey – does offer many benefits, particularly for comparing the views of different groups or establishing the strength of a view. However, many priority-setting exercises involving the public would benefit from using a combination of quantitative and qualitative approaches.

Quantitative methods

Surveys

Surveys, especially those using structured questionnaires, can provide a systematic approach to measurement of a specific issue. They are systematic in that all data are

---

Box 5.3:   Some methods of 'involving' the public in the NHS

- Surveys with self-completion questionnaires:
    with random samples
    with haphazard or opportunistic samples
- Interview surveys (structured or semi-structured questionnaires):
    with random samples
    with haphazard or opportunistic samples
- Indepth interviews
- Observation
- Rapid appraisal approaches
- Focus groups
- Panels (one-off or continuing)
- Citizens' juries
- Liaison with user groups
- Questionnaires or reply forms in local/HA newspapers, leaflets, etc.
- Press releases and advertisements
- Suggestions/complaints boxes/slips
- Public meetings
- Public representatives on decision-making bodies

---

collected in a standardised way, thus allowing for the aggregation of views from different individuals within the sample surveyed. Importantly, this process of aggregation allows for comparisons to be made between various groups of respondents such that differences of view can be made clear and potentially accommodated in subsequent decision making. The aggregation of the information derived from the survey questions allows a common base to be established and hence changes in views, perhaps resulting from a health authority initiative to provide additional information about a particular service, to be monitored over time. Possibly, though, the most important contribution of all is that a properly conducted sample survey allows conclusions to be made about the population from which it is drawn.

Selecting the sample

The process of selecting survey respondents is, of course, vital in the context of priority setting, as the earlier discussion of representativeness illustrated. Random sampling is necessary to enable generalisation from the findings of a sample survey to the whole of the relevant population – the target population. However, pure random samples (where every individual member of the target population has an equal chance of being selected), which are also sufficiently large to allow generalisations to be made, may be difficult to achieve because of inadequate definition of the target population, deficiencies in the population-based sampling frames available and difficulties in making contact with certain groups of the population.

Further, the large number of defining characteristics – taxpayer, citizen, healthcare user, carer, age, etc. – which may influence the views of any individual about health service provision may make it difficult to obtain a suitably 'representative' random sample. Large stratified samples, where the size of the sample drawn from each stratum is in proportion to the size of that stratum, could be used to cope with this problem. However, in the resulting analysis, care needs to be taken to avoid producing an averaging type of response which denies the possibility of smaller subgroups being able to advocate their view. Disproportionate stratified sampling (where smaller strata may be deliberately oversampled) allows the voice of minority groups within the community to be heard but again there is the danger of one group cancelling out the views of another. With disproportionate sampling, care also, of course, has to be taken to ensure appropriate weighting of response where a population-wide result is a requirement.

Some surveys use convenience, haphazard or self-selecting samples. However, even where a large number of responses are obtained, such surveys do not enable generalisations and conclusions to be drawn about the views of the relevant population as a whole.

Structured versus semi-structured questionnaires

Surveys, especially those using structured self-completion questionnaires, are particularly useful for providing, quite quickly, relatively cost-effective but relatively superficial snapshots of the views of a group in terms of their behaviour, their beliefs, their attitudes and their preferences. Surveys are less good when very complex issues are involved and where the views are not based on respondents' direct experience but rather are about projected events or experiences, which is of course where the priority-setting process requires the focus to be located.

The detailed conduct of the survey is also an issue in terms of effective engagement of the public in priority setting. The questionnaire may vary in its degree of structure. The more structured the questionnaire, the easier it is to answer and analyse. A lot of very good data can be collected if the issues lend themselves to this degree of pre-structure. The difficulty, however, is that such structure requires a very clear set of prior categories of potential responses, which acts to restrict greatly the range and variability of views gathered. Essentially, the cognitive structure of the investigator is imposed upon the measure and respondents are forced to provide their individual thoughts within this restricted, externally derived framework. Such structured measures are more appropriate for routine information issues.

Where the situation requires that the respondent be allowed more flexibility, unstructured approaches, which often require an interview, may be used. In this instance some questions can be framed but others left open for further probing and elaboration. This will probably involve face-to-face or possibly telephone interviews. Whilst this allows for greater exploration and follow-up of complex aspects of the questionnaire, the reality is that such interviewing processes are costly in terms of time and resources. Typically smaller samples are utilised with this approach although, as a result, the generalisability of the findings may be jeopardised. Interviewers require good training to avoid bias but the method is certainly of value where the topic is complex and dynamic and the likely outcome relatively unknown.

The degree of public engagement is a significant issue here. The face-to-face interview requires a considerable degree of prior contact and logistic support in order to place interviewer and interviewee at the right location at the right time. It also requires a willingness on behalf of those to be interviewed either to allow someone to visit them or to travel to a pre-arranged meeting. The extra effort will interact with the issue of representativeness. Why will some people agree to meet an interviewer to discuss future health services? Do they have a special interest in the topic? Have they had a 'bad' experience and want to tell someone? Are those who opt out similar in views to those who participate – and do we know? Volunteers may well be different from those who do not volunteer. As with all surveys, it is important in the conduct of face-to-face interviews to establish whatever information is possible about the non-responders to see if there appears to be a systematic difference between them and responders and hence possibly a difference in views held.

The questionnaire which is distributed for self-completion avoids some of the dynamic aspects of potential bias. However, because it is a more impersonal process it is typically affected by a lower response rate and hence a larger set of unknown non-respondents. Response rates to self-completion questionnaires can be very variable. The covering letter, the nature of the organisation conducting the survey and the offer of incentives can all have an effect (Campanelli, 1995). Whilst follow-up reminders are of value, one of the key factors in overall response rate seems to be the perceived value of the topic of the questionnaire. Is it seen as relevant and important? Do respondents feel their replies may have an impact upon something they value? The priority-setting context seems less assured in terms of these influences. Certainly the topic of priority setting is accepted as important but the legitimacy of the process is less clear (Lomas, 1997).

Constructing questionnaires

How can we conduct a survey to facilitate the collection of the best data possible? There are sets of good-practice principles about the construction of questionnaires, such as sound piloting, clear layout, attention to the language and the level of literacy of potential respondents. But, in the context of priority setting, two areas are crucial: (a) the attention paid to the exact wording and meaning of the questions; and (b) the nature of the scaling construction used to assess the responses given, which is covered in more detail in the following chapter.

In terms of the wording of questionnaires concerned with priority setting, a few general points should be noted. It is unwise to invite respondents to engage immediately with a complex set of resource allocation and 'hard choice' decisions. Therefore, a set of so-called 'funnel' questions is probably worthwhile, whereby the general topic area is introduced and the respondent is made to feel at ease by being able to deal with quite simple, clear questions. Gradually more taxing and demanding questions may be introduced but at least a relevant mindset will have been created.

Decisions relating to conflicting priorities in the delivery of healthcare are, almost by definition, complex. It is therefore rather difficult in a structured questionnaire, especially one intended for self-completion, to adhere to the principles of simple questions without jargon or without the need for specific knowledge. Funnel questions are important to establish the respondent's awareness of the context and, in this instance, perhaps to define more precisely their awareness of 'health issues' such as direct or indirect experience of particular services, current health status, etc. Within this, care must be taken to avoid leading questions such that respondents appear to be guided towards a seemingly inevitable position – possibly that envisaged by the author of the questionnaire. Priority-setting measures may be especially vulnerable to the issue of social desirability, i.e. where respondents provide the answers they perceive the investigator would like to hear. Questions relating to priority conflicts between drug addicts, the mentally disturbed and, for example, premature babies need very careful handling.

In terms of the type of response mode to be used in questionnaires, a great variety of scales exist. These are discussed in depth in Chapter Six and in the Appendix. It is especially important to make a clear distinction between rating scales and ranking procedures as they are widely used but frequently confused. The latter approach requires individual respondents to place various options in an order so that the item placed first is deemed to be most important or most significant, depending upon the dimension being considered. All subsequent items are then placed in descending order. Rating scales, by contrast, require that each item (question) be rated on a scale. The commonly used Likert Scale typically contains up to five points, so that a score of 1 might mean one completely disagrees with the question and 5 equates to total agreement. The visual analogue scale (VAS) presents respondents with a single line to represent the score options, anchored at each end by a relatively extreme position such as 'best' or 'worst'. The respondent places a cross on the line at a position reflecting their view of a particular question. This process has the effect of removing the numerical equivalent which seems to act as a constraint since, with the analogue scale, respondents tend to provide a greater diversity of view. A full description of these methods is presented in the Appendix.

The survey approach in action

The survey approach, utilising various types of questionnaire, has been employed by a number of health authorities in their efforts to involve the public in priority setting (see Chapter Seven). Tensions between lay and professional views are evident in some of the findings. For example, in response to a questionnaire distributed by Bath Health Authority which achieved a 50% response rate, the public overwhelmingly endorsed kidney dialysis (81%) but far less so family planning (23%). They also strongly supported the retention of 12 community hospitals, in contrast to the views of the health authority. The conclusion reached was that the public needed more information to support their involvement in priority setting but that questionnaires did offer a useful way of establishing public views (Richardson *et al.*, 1992). Similar conflict between the public and professionals was reported by Mid-Essex Health Authority. Once again the conclusion was that the public needs more information (Lutton, 1992). Whilst this view is almost certainly valid, it does suggest, at least to the cynical mind, that the public need more information until they get it right, i.e. agree with the professional view.

In contrast, Solihull Health Authority used a questionnaire with 630 adult residents and ultimately obtained a satisfactory response rate after three reminders and personal visits. Eleven specific health services were rank ordered against two contrasting scenarios – one where the health authority was losing money and one where it was gaining. The questionnaire responses and rankings were consistent and were close to those of the purchaser, perhaps because indicative cost information had also been provided. However, the process was clearly time consuming and expensive and it is not clear how far it has subsequently influenced purchasing decisions.

Facilitated meetings

Public meetings are the traditional and perhaps rather anachronistic method of health authorities offering plans and intentions to public scrutiny. The cost, poor attendance and vulnerability of such meetings to lobby groups have been well documented (Edwards, 1995). However, there have been attempts to structure and facilitate large meetings, often with audiences selected according to some notion of representativeness.

An example of a very structured approach to obtaining quantitative information from meetings comes from the United States as a development from the 'Just Caring' project, which among other things aimed to articulate 'a set of basic social values' and 'a set of principles for priority-setting among health care needs' (Fleck, 1992, pp.1631–2). Fleck developed a 3–4-hour community education programme (with shorter variants) which since 1991 has been addressed to at least 100 audiences (professionals as well as community leaders and the lay public), each of 100–150 people. As part of the programme, the audience are invited to respond to a series of statements (moral judgements and policy options) using keypads linked by radio frequency to a notebook computer, which can instantly aggregate up to 250 responses. The statements, to which the permitted responses are (1) Strongly Agree, (2) Agree, (3) Uncertain, (4) Disagree, (5) Strongly Disagree, come out of a scenario (presented on video) that raises a specific rationing/resource allocation issue. Graphs, showing the responses in bar chart format, are displayed and discussed during the session, eliciting their reasons for their judgements from audience members who gave different responses. Keypads are unique so, although the individual identity of each respondent is unknown, questions on gender, age, race/ethnicity and professional background enable the responses to be analysed by any of these categories. The resulting graphs are produced in hard-copy format after each session (Fleck, 1995a; Fleck and Hogan, 1993).

Qualitative methods

Qualitative methods, by their nature, have a different orientation and outcome from the more quantitative approaches. They are broadly concerned with the experience and meaning of events as seen by the participant. Thus, they are more geared towards answering questions about why something happened or why people feel or behave in particular ways. Qualitative methods can produce this greater depth of understanding. Sensitive issues and minority views can be revealed using such techniques.

The difficulties associated with qualitative methods relate primarily to the concept of reliability and the degree to which an indepth account or view from a restricted number of individuals can be used as the basis for more generalised and representative decisions. Nonetheless, qualitative methods have proved attractive in the context of priority setting as investigators have begun to recognise the deficiencies in seeking direct quantitative outcomes or decisions from the public. Individual values can be explored in depth using qualitative techniques so that bodies such as health authorities can be guided in the way they make decisions about health priorities by their awareness of the public's fundamental position.

Indepth interviews

The most obvious qualitative research method is the indepth interview with a single individual. Whilst of value in general, it has not been used to any great extent in priority setting since it clearly confronts the issue of generalisability in a most extreme form. However, along with several other methods which have emerged in this area, including focus groups, citizens' juries and rapid appraisal techniques which are discussed below, indepth interviews can be usefully employed in conjunction with quantitative techniques, in particular to assist in the framing of questions.

Focus groups

Focus groups may be thought of as a loosely planned conversation with a small group of people, typically 8–12 participants. The group is facilitated, often by the investigator, hence the notion of 'planning' to ensure that the group addresses the critical topics. But this planning can be very light with groups encouraged to explore the issue as widely as they like and in whatever direction seems appropriate. The focus group provides, by sharing, exploring and contrasting the ideas in greater depth and breadth, fuller coverage of issues than is possible in a series of individual interviews with an equivalent number of people (Kitzinger, 1996). Discussion can be supplemented by small tasks, such as allocating some aspect of a health authority budget. In this way indepth discussion, allowing information exchange to occur, can be linked to a more direct decision-making process.

Typically focus groups have been used to examine a specific issue and often this prescribes the type of people one wishes to participate in the group, i.e. teenagers might be recruited to examine views about family planning or sexual health. Some would argue that this is an appropriate use of focus groups – single issue and homogeneous membership. In the context of priority setting, however, depending on the purpose of the exercise, this homogeneity of membership may create a problem. If the teenagers, say, advocate increased expenditure on health promotion with regard to contraception, this might well be contrasted with a group of pensioners who endorse more expenditure on continuing care. The health authority in receipt of such views simply knows that groups of people, as opposed to individuals, differ. A compromise decision may satisfy neither group and a decision in one direction appears to disregard the views of one of the groups. However, if the decisions under consideration concern the setting of priorities within and between services for teenagers, a focus group consisting solely of teenagers might be entirely appropriate.

Generally, focus groups have been used to explore people's views and experiences of various groups about a specific condition, service or treatment. For instance, in another context Milman (1993) used focus groups on the choice of holiday destination. Further, the limited time involved in a focus group ($1^1/_2$–2 hours) and the problem of representativeness have limited their usage in directly setting wider health priorities.

Standing panels

Attempts to provide continuity and/or overcome perceived problems of lack of knowledge have led to the assembling of 'standing' groups of consumers, who can be engaged in consultation over a period of time. These can range from a few dozen people, who constitute one or more focus groups who meet periodically (as described above), to a standing panel of 1000 or more local residents, who are invited to complete questionnaires from time to time.

Hoinville and Courtenay (1979, p.173) describe experimenting with 'community panels' – small groups of eight people, meeting several times to learn about, discuss and evaluate policies.* One of their first uses of such groups was in South Yorkshire, where 64 members of the public constituted eight groups, which each met on three

---

* They suggest that these are similar to Murray and Berrill's (1975) Citizen Feedback Project, where some panels met up to ten times in a six-week period for lengthy discussions.

occasions. They suggest that the quality of the discussion falls off as groups grow above eight people. They point to the danger of such groups that, as with any 'jury', some members can dominate but claim that they have an advantage over traditional juries in that discussion can be controlled and steered by a trained researcher.

Taking the idea of standing panels further, Meddin *et al.* (1990) describe a sophisticated Health Advisory Network, set up in Western Australia and consisting of both consumers and providers of health services, to provide advice on the planning, policy and administration of the state's health services and to serve as a forum for health issues.

Fleck (1992, p.1630) describes proposals for a consensus-building project in Michigan which, for a variety of reasons, did not move beyond the pilot stage (Fleck, 1995a). The project was intended to involve 20–25 sites, each with 50 project participants. Each site would hold 25–30 public forums over a two-year period in which those 50 individuals would participate. The public would be invited to attend, reading packs would be supplied to participants and university staff would serve as facilitators.

As an even more ambitious proposal, and predicated on the existence of a single comprehensive health plan for the US, Fleck (1992, pp.1624–5) outlined his vision of district health councils, one per congressional district, each made up of 50 citizen/patients who would be 'representative' but would not represent any special interest. Each district council would elect its 'most judicious and fair-minded' member to serve on a national health congress. That congress would establish an issue agenda for all district councils. 'What would emerge from the democratic deliberation at the district level would be a local consensus that would provide the partially refined material for a national consensus.'

Citizens' juries

Citizens' jury methodology developed in the USA and Germany over the last 20 years but has recently attracted the attention of the UK health service as a method of securing 'informed' participation (Coote and Lenaghan, 1997; Stewart *et al.*, 1994). A typical pattern to a citizens' jury involves the recruitment of 10–20 'citizens', who meet over several days. They are presented with verbal and written material relevant to the topic to be considered. In some cases, 'jurors' are able to call their own witnesses and request the provision of additional written material. A moderator helps the jury members to utilise the material and a consensus report with recommendations, 'the verdict', is produced.

A number of pilot citizens' jury projects have been conducted and some have been evaluated (McIver, 1998). Broadly positive outcomes were observed in terms of the ability and willingness of jurors to engage themselves with the materials and decisions to be made. However, it was felt that, despite the semantic connotation of a jury, the role of such activities is to influence rather than determine priorities. The health authorities were positive too about how the juries had enabled the public (at least

those on the jury) to understand complex health issues and to make useful recommendations. They were, however, less enthusiastic about some of the processes
involved in citizens' juries, notably the considerable planning and lead time required
to prepare for a jury and the considerable expense (preparation, paying jurors, venue,
etc.) as they were found to be much more expensive than other methods. Perhaps the
most important issue was the time and effort needed to recruit a relatively small
number of local people whilst recognising that such a group may not have any
commitment or legitimacy as viewed by the wider population.

Other concerns related to the degree to which complex issues were fully understood
and the degree to which it might be possible for the health authority to manipulate the
evidence presented and thereby influence the outcome. Finally, there remained the
continuing dilemma as to whether the recommendations should be viewed as interesting and potentially influential advice or more as a binding decision on the health
authority.

Another concern that might be raised in connection with citizens' juries relates to
their name, which appears to attempt to draw legitimacy from the analogy with legal
juries. However, the parallels could be misleading. First, legal juries are charged with
determining the (positive) facts of a case, not with presenting their own, informed or
uninformed (normative) values. Second, over the centuries, as citizens (or subjects),
we have *de facto* delegated our role in the legal process to juries and it is from this that
they enjoy popular legitimacy. No such delegation, *de facto* or not, exists in the case of
citizens' juries. Indeed, it is interesting to note that in Germany the term 'planning
cells' is used; the name 'citizens' juries' was coined and patented in the USA (Stewart,
1995).

Clayton (1998, p.59) also questions the analogy with legal juries, but extends his
argument to question the whole rationale of public participation in priority setting.

*Should they [citizens' juries] be viewed on the model of standard juries, in which an
independently fair result is thought to obtain (conviction for the guilty and acquittal for
the innocent) and jury participation is judged to be the best available means of securing
that outcome? Or, should they be defended in terms of eliciting the population's informed
preferences about priority setting? Plainly, this relates to the central issue of whether
justice in the distribution of health care is a matter on which the people may legitimately
vote or, like the franchise, a matter which is just or unjust independently of the majority's preference ... the questions which such juries address must be restricted to those
on which the public are competent and entitled to speak ...*

Despite the various misgivings, it does seem likely that the basic jury approach will be
explored further, perhaps with modification to the current model to accommodate
feedback from the evaluation report.

Public meetings

Although, as discussed earlier, using the traditional method of public meetings to offer health authority plans and intentions to public scrutiny can be criticised on grounds of cost, poor attendance (except where proposals to close a hospital are under consideration) and vulnerability to lobby groups, there have been some imaginative attempts to make meetings more useful. For instance, some health authorities have 'invited' local groups (community, social, religious, etc.) to organise meetings at which HA representatives present their case.

Rapid appraisal

Another increasingly popular approach, drawing on methodologies created for use in developing countries, is rapid appraisal (Ong and Humphris, 1994 *inter alia*). This approach is based on the notion that approximately 30 key people in a community can be interviewed in depth to derive a representative picture of the views, priorities or needs of that community. Sometimes the participants are selected from a wider meeting called to discuss health issues. The 'key' people selected to participate typically might represent three subgroups such as a professional group (local GP, nurse, teacher, etc.), those seen as community leaders (parish councillors, voluntary organisation leaders) and members of the ordinary public deemed to be in touch with local opinion (shopkeepers, publicans, etc.). Some rapid appraisals have also involved a discussion within this key group and an attempt to rank order different competing health issues, with feedback to the original wider community about the deliberations and the outcome from the key group members.

Clearly, the method has some element of community involvement and is frequently advocated as a catalyst to future community initiatives rather than as a direct decision-making process. Sefton Health Authority conducted a rapid appraisal which typified this concept. Discrepancies were identified between the various sub-groupings and, on the basis of trying to explore and resolve the differences, communication between the public and local health and government bodies was said to have improved (Ong *et al.*, 1991). Other rapid appraisals have been undertaken to address the issue of community needs and the findings generally illustrate the public's view of need as broader than health – involving clean streets, leisure provision, lighting, etc. Whilst useful and important, these are still some way from the specific 'hard choice' decisions implied in current conceptions of priority setting.

Repertory grid

The repertory grid method is an approach designed specifically to understand the respondent's views of particular issues but in the language of the respondent rather than that of the investigator. In this method, different stimuli (health interventions or treatments) are presented in a three-way comparison, known as the triad method, and respondents are asked to say how two of the stimuli are alike but different from the third. This process is repeated several times and in this way the respondent's 'constructs' (or the way in which they see the world) are elicited. These constructs therefore indicate how people might think about various topics and the constructs, being those of the public, can then be used in a rating grid with a larger set of the public to examine how they feel about a specific issue. Such a method could be helpful in trying to establish fundamental public values about various competing healthcare priorities.

Vignettes or scenarios

A method gaining some support in the priority-setting area is that of scenarios or vignettes. These are essentially short descriptions of situations setting a context for the particular question within the overall description. The attraction of such an approach with priority-setting type issues is its potential to provide the public with sufficient information, for example treatment cost or outcome, to make a decision. However, such scenarios are difficult to write without giving even a minor hint as to the 'appropriate' direction of the answer and they therefore must be used with care. Further, the 'rule of rescue', discussed in Chapter Four, may mean that the values revealed in respect of the 'identified' individuals typically used in such vignettes are different from the values revealed in connection with 'statistical' (unidentified) individuals. Further, vignettes tend to concentrate on individual inter-patient comparisons, which may not be the appropriate arena for public involvement.

How do methods of engaging the public compare?

This chapter has attempted to consider some of the conceptual issues around engaging the public in the process of priority setting. Doubts have been raised about the appropriateness and democratic legitimacy of this process, especially at the most extreme 'hard choice' end of the dimension where some types of care are restricted in order to ensure access to others (see Chapter Eight). However, efforts to involve the public have proceeded and some of the principal methods of engagement have been described.

Large-scale surveys, based on random sampling, have the advantage of providing some statistically valid basis for decision making and perhaps offer the greatest degree of representativeness amongst the methods. They also offer the advantage of being able to explore the clear differences between sub-groups in the population. However, they are of necessity a simplification of complex issues and cannot cope well with demands for further information or indeed any uncertainty experienced by respondents in the decisions made. They therefore risk producing a spurious certainty in outcome. Equally, the averaged outcome of numerical data can represent the lowest and least satisfactory denominator.

Qualitative methods, by contrast, do allow for this exploration of complex issues and suggest that, with appropriate support, the public can, and in many instances are willing to, make difficult decisions. The fundamental problem of such approaches, though, relates to generalisability, representativeness and legitimacy.

Rutt (1997) examined the three different methods (rapid appraisal, focus groups and surveys) in practice within a research study and reports variation in outcome which may well be related to the method chosen. If such findings are repeated then the choice of approach for engaging the public in priority setting becomes a critical issue, which needs to be assessed thoroughly before action is taken to implement decisions based on information which may be an artefact of the method used to elicit that information. Ultimately, which method, or combination of methods, is most appropriate in any given circumstance will depend on the objectives or purpose of the exercise.

CHAPTER SIX

Eliciting values for priority setting

Priority setting involves values. Whose values should be involved – those of the public, users, politicians, authority or board members, managers and/or professionals – is, as seen in earlier chapters, a matter of some debate. Nevertheless, values are involved in numerous areas of priority setting in healthcare, including the following.

- Valuing different health states, often in order to construct some form of health status index or QALY. The resulting scales can then be used to value health improvements from different treatments. When combined with cost information, such information can produce QALY league tables.
- Valuing or choosing between different patient groups (e.g. old versus young, men versus women, deserving versus non-deserving) (Mooney *et al.*, 1995).
- Directly valuing or choosing between different health service areas or between different treatments.
- Valuing attributes of health, health services and/or treatments, usually to use them as evaluation or weighting criteria in a two-stage process.
- Valuing or choosing between methods of healthcare delivery (e.g. treatment at home versus treatment in hospital, etc.).
- Valuing preferences in healthcare delivery (e.g. appointment systems versus open surgeries, food, decor, etc.).

Unlike implicit priority setting, where the values involved usually remain unarticu-lated, explicit priority setting generally requires that values and preferences are elicited explicitly. Techniques for eliciting values and preferences have a long history in several disciplines, including economics, operational research, psychology and political science. Some of the techniques and methodologies are particularly or even uniquely suited to one of the areas listed above but many are appropriate for a wide range of uses. Further, most of the techniques for eliciting values from users and the public in general are equally relevant for eliciting values and preferences from professionals and authority members.

As noted above, techniques for eliciting values and preferences have a long history in several disciplines. The different disciplines, however, tend to seek models and methods of value elicitation which are grounded within their own disciplinary theory. This can lead to problems both because of a general lack of cross-disciplinary fertilisation and because techniques from other disciplines may be judged to lack theoretical validity. However, whilst acknowledging the wish of many disciplines to remain within the confines of their own theories, it is worth noting that theoretical validity and purity do not always coincide with acceptability, people's comprehension and even people's value systems.

A further danger of straying into a cross-disciplinary area is the difficulty, especially in a short space, of synthesising the arguments, theories and techniques of such disparate disciplines. The impossibility of mastering all the contemporary debates in all the different disciplines and sub-areas means some of the discussion here will inevitably appear lacking or even naïve to some disciplinary experts. The reader is advised to consult the literature within their chosen discipline to obtain a full understanding of the theoretical considerations from that viewpoint. The aim here is to extract and propose practical and acceptable methodologies, which are appropriate for use in the health service and which do not raise too many theoretical objections.

It is important to ensure a correct balance between theoretical validity and user acceptability. In particular, how far we should move in favour of the latter and away from the former requires careful consideration. At the very least, however, users of a technique should understand the values implicit within that technique, the form of choice being imposed on respondents, the implications of the aggregation of individual values and the relevance/appropriateness of the chosen techniques to the purposes of their particular application. Basically, the methods selected should be doing what the 'researchers' (users) and, in most cases, the participants/respondents think they are doing; thus transparency is an important criterion.

There is clear evidence both from the literature and from the survey of health authorities reported in Chapter Seven that there is considerable reinvention of the wheel. Many projects within the NHS demonstrate little or no evidence of awareness of the literature or of experience elsewhere. However, it is interesting to note that this is by no means a new phenomenon: in the 1970s Huber (1974, p.1393) observed that:

On many occasions management scientists conscientiously expend considerable time and thought in developing MAU [multi-attribute utility] models, i.e. re-inventing the wheel rather than just making minor modifications to fit a particular situation.

Issues in value elicitation

A large number of issues arise in connection with eliciting values and preferences and using these within decision making. Many decisions within health services are multi-criteria or multi-attribute, rather than the more straightforward single criterion or single attribute. Some approaches assume a linear relationship between quantity and value (i.e. 'value' increases in proportion to the amount of resource provided, service produced or numbers treated), whilst others accommodate a non-linear relationship (usually diminishing returns, with 'value' increasing more slowly than resources, services or treatments). Some approaches to eliciting values incorporate risk or uncertainty which, whilst it may have relevance to individual decisions taken in the face of uncertainty, may not be necessary, or even appropriate, when addressing policy decisions. Most approaches elicit values from individuals but then seek to aggregate those values to produce group or societal values. These issues are addressed in more detail below.

Single-stage versus multistage decisions

Nearly all (perhaps all) decisions which arise within healthcare policy involve multiple objectives. Thus many approaches and models are two- or multi-stage (multi-attribute or multi-criterion), valuing first the attributes/criteria and then the options against those criteria. In many instances the criteria or attributes are valued explicitly as a separate stage of the decision process. However, some methods value the criteria/attributes implicitly, determining or inferring their values from observations of choices between options possessing different 'degrees' of the different attributes. The former approach is far more transparent to the user but can be limited where there is a complex relationship between different attributes/criteria.

Many methods use a single-stage process, even when valuing options that clearly possess multiple attributes. Thus, respondents are asked to choose directly between treatments, between packages of care or between different services. In other cases, respondents are asked to value attributes such as access, waiting times, friendliness of staff, etc. without the resulting values being formally incorporated into a two-stage model, although presumably the values so obtained will be taken into account informally within the decision-making process.

Many, if not most, explicit methods of eliciting values are applicable both to single-stage models and to the individual stages of multistage models. Implicit methods are usually associated with multistage models although it could be argued that implicit and explicit methods converge in single-stage models.

Constrained (forced choice) versus unconstrained valuations

Most explicit methods of eliciting values can be divided between those methods which require respondents to make constrained (or forced) choices, which 'incorporate some notion of sacrifice' (Shackley and Ryan, 1995, p.198), and those which allow unconstrained choices or valuations. The latter are characterised by scaling or rating methods, where each criterion/attribute/option is valued independently of the others (although the effect of constrained choice can be obtained by subsequent normalisation – rescaling each participant's responses so that they total to a fixed sum across the competing criteria/attributes/options). Constrained choices involve some form of trade-off between different attributes/criteria or alternatives and include a wide range of voting, ranking, comparison and trade-off techniques.

However, technically, the difference is sometimes more apparent than real, with some techniques acting as hybrids and, in any case, the potential to normalise noted above. The relevance of offering respondents unconstrained rather than constrained choices can lie more in psychological effect on the respondent. Generally, however, if the attributes or options to be valued are independent and not in competition, unconstrained methods are preferable. Where they are in competition, and especially where that fact is important to the purposes of the exercise, constrained methods are to be preferred.

However, depending on the purpose of the exercise, even where options are in competition, unconstrained choices may be appropriate. Consider, for example, a health centre with development funds sufficient for either a ramp for wheelchair access or a play area. If user involvement is viewed as a 'voting' exercise, it may well be appropriate to use a method which gives a wheelchair-bound woman with small children the same constrained choice between the schemes as an able-bodied man without children. On the other hand, if the aim of the user 'involvement' is to determine the relative importance to users of the competing schemes in order to inform decision making, an unconstrained choice (such as scaling or rating), which allows the woman to give a high score to both and the man a low score to both, would appear appropriate, despite any resulting inter-respondent inequity when the ratings are aggregated, as will be discussed later.

Technical considerations can also intrude. Mutually exclusive attributes or options can place severe limitations on many methodologies offering constrained choices. Unconstrained (non-normalised) valuations can cause problems (especially inter-person equity) in aggregation, over and above the general problems posed by aggregation discussed below.

Aggregation of individual values

The issue of the aggregation of individual values poses possibly insoluble ethical and technical problems. At the simplest ethical level, is it legitimate to combine one person's rating of 10 with another's rating of 0 for the same item and conclude that, on average, the group or societal rating of that item is 5? At the very least, this may 'lead to an unnecessary "flattening out" of public opinion' (Donovan and Coast, 1996, p.227). Should, indeed, majority preferences be permitted to over-rule minority preferences? In addition, technical problems abound. As a result, viewpoints range from the stance that it is impossible to make interpersonal comparisons of utility and thus aggregating values across individuals is impermissible, to the argument that societal choices have to be made (using voting in elections as an example) so we should stop arguing and simply add up the individual values.

The theoretical considerations relating to the aggregation of individual preferences have been a major preoccupation of the, sometimes abstruse, social choice theory and public choice literature going back over 200 years. A classic problem of aggregating preferences is demonstrated by Condorcet's *voting paradox*. This shows that the aggregation of transitive preferences of individuals can yield intransitive 'group' preferences. That is, even if each individual has transitive preferences, i.e. if they prefer x to y and y to z, then they prefer x to z, it is possible, when the individual preferences are aggregated, that the group preferences are intransitive (see Box 6.1), i.e. the group prefers x to y, y to z, but prefers z to x (Brown and Jackson, 1978, pp.72–4; Enelow, 1997, p.149). For practical purposes in the health service, this paradox is only likely to cause serious problems where values are very heterogeneous, in particular where diametrically opposed views are held, for instance in connection with abortion.

Box 6.1:   Voting paradox

Let us assume three 'voters', Tom, Dick and Harry, and three options, Amber, Blue and Claret. Each voter's preference order is transitive, as shown below.

	Tom	*Dick*	*Harry*
First choice	Amber	Blue	Claret
Second choice	Blue	Claret	Amber
Third choice	Claret	Amber	Blue

In an election between Amber and Blue only, Amber will win
In an election between Blue and Claret only, Blue will win
In an election between Amber and Claret only, Claret will win

Thus the group's preferences are:

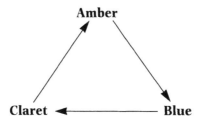

Arrow's *impossibility theorem** (Arrow, 1963) 'is the most celebrated impossibility theorem in the literature on social choice theory' (Pattanaik, 1997, p.205). It shows that there is no way to aggregate individual choices that satisfies a set of minimum conditions and axioms, which include transitivity, non-dictatorship (there is no individual whose preferences are imposed as the societal preferences) and the weak Pareto criterion (if all individuals prefer *x* to *y*, then society must prefer *x* to *y*) (Arrow, 1963; Bonner, 1986, pp.58–71; McLean, 1987, pp.165–8, 172–6; Pattanaik, 1997). However, possibly of greatest interest in the health service, given the proliferation of ranking exercises, is Arrow's Condition 3 – *the independence of irrelevant alternatives*. This requires that the preference ordering of a set of alternatives is unaffected by the addition (or subtraction) of an 'irrelevant' alternative, i.e. if A is preferred to B and B is preferred to C, the introduction of an 'irrelevant' alternative D should not alter the ABC ordering, wherever D itself is placed in the ordering. It is easy to demonstrate how this condition can be violated when rank positions are used as scores and summed (see Box 6.2).

This should not be dismissed simply as theoretical game playing. Ranking is used widely within the health service for eliciting values or preferences and, in many instances, the rank positions are used as 'scores' and summed. The potential for manipulating results, whether intentionally or inadvertently, by including *irrelevant* options must be recognised.

Thus, not only can the method of eliciting preferences yield different values, the choice of aggregation method can affect the result. As Weale (1990, p.122) points out: 'The same set of preferences in a community amalgamated by a difference voting rule will yield a different collective choice'. It is this fact that leads to the heated debates on replacing first-past-the-post voting with some form of proportional representation.

Thus, at the very least, users of techniques should be aware of the dangers of aggregation and of the implications of different methods. Perez (1994), agreeing that there is no truly satisfactory procedure for the aggregation of preferences in ordinal contexts, suggests that a framework should be devised to help choose a relatively good rule for a given situation. Further, in view of the many problems associated with aggregation, there is often a case for avoiding single aggregated measures and presenting the full range of responses. Such an approach is commonly associated with Delphi exercises where individual responses are mapped on to a bar chart or histogram. Figure 6.1 shows this approach adapted to present respondents' scores for three different options, all of which have a mean 'score' of 5 (out of 10), but with very different distributions of respondent scores contributing to that mean.

Another problem of aggregation relates to equity between respondents. Even the concept of equality or equity in decision making is not without problems. Rae and Schickler (1997, p.165) point out that at a basic level, given two individuals with differing preferences, 'any workable decision rule embodies some seed of inequality',

---

* Although it is normally known as Arrow's *impossibility theorem*, Arrow (1963) names it the *possibility theorem*.

Box 6.2:   Independence of irrelevant alternatives

Let us assume four 'voters', Tom, Dick, Harry and Joe, and four options, Amber, Blue, Claret and Dun. Each voter ranks the options from 1 to 4 in order of preference, as shown below. Then the rank positions for each option are summed giving a total score (and the mean rank position calculated). This gives the group's ranking of the options in the order: Amber, Blue, Claret and Dun.

	Tom	Dick	Harry	Joe	Total 'score'	Mean 'score'	Group ranking
Amber	1	1	2	1	5	1.25	1
Blue	4	2	1	3	10	2.50	2
Claret	2	4	4	2	12	3.00	3
Dun	3	3	3	4	13	3.25	4

A new *irrelevant* option, Violet, is introduced and each voter includes it in their ranking, as shown below.

	Tom	Dick	Harry	Joe	Total 'score'	Mean 'score'	Group ranking
Amber	1	1	2	2	6	1.50	1
Blue	5	2	1	4	12	3.00	2
Claret	2	5	5	3	15	3.75	5
Dun	3	3	3	5	14	3.50	4
Violet	4	4	4	1	13	3.25	3

However, although the inclusion of Violet did not cause any voter to alter the relative rank positions of Amber, Blue, Claret and Dun, the aggregated group ranking is now Amber, Blue, Violet, Dun and Claret, i.e. the group now 'prefers' Dun to Claret but before the introduction of Violet, the group 'preferred' Claret to Dun.

The same result is observed if reverse 'scores' are used, with the highest ranked option receiving the highest 'score'.

and they go on to discuss a number of equity criteria. For our purposes here, however, inter-respondent equity requires simply that respondents have equal 'voting' power – equal weight – in any aggregated values. This does not rule out the use of inter-respondent *inequity*. There may well be, in some circumstances, justification for allowing, or even allocating, different respondents different weights in the aggregated values, for instance if it is decided to give greater weight to the views of members of some disadvantaged group – but it would seem preferable that such unequal weights are incorporated explicitly rather than inequality being an accidental outcome of the methodology. Further, as noted above, by the definition of equity proposed here, the case of the wheelchair-bound woman with children and the able-bodied man with no

Option 1

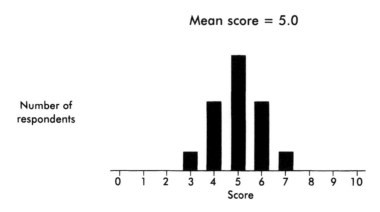

Option 2

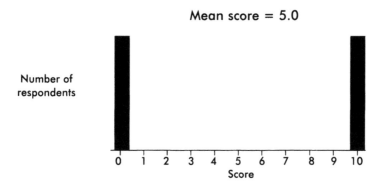

Option 3

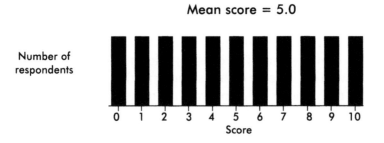

Figure 6.1 Results presented using the Delphi approach.

children could result in inter-respondent inequity if a non-normalised, unconstrained method is used to elicit preferences for the competing schemes.

Aggregation is also affected by individuals not revealing their true preferences by strategic voting, co-operating or trading votes, as in 'logrolling' (Mueller, 1997, p.12) and game playing (prisoner's dilemma), or by 'reverse engineering' the decision methodology to ensure their desired outcome is achieved (French and Stewart, 1993).

Although we need methodologies which can be used to inform priority setting within health services and thus need techniques which are sufficiently simple and robust for widespread use and which are able to incorporate the values of large numbers of individuals, it is important not to ignore the practical and theoretical problems associated with aggregation. Further, it should be noted that much of social choice theory is concerned with aggregation of ordinal preferences, often with the (relatively limited) objective of determining an overall winner or, especially in the case of Arrow's impossibility theorem, with the objective of achieving societal ordinal preferences. However, many applications associated with valuing health states and priority setting within healthcare require, or at least use, cardinal valuations from individuals and seek to aggregate these into collective or societal cardinal valuations or utilities.

Overview of techniques for eliciting preferences/values

As mentioned above, there are a large number of methods, derived from a variety of disciplines, for eliciting, either explicitly or implicitly, values and preferences from individuals and for aggregating such values. Some of the techniques found in the literature, with greater or lesser degrees of theoretical justification, and/or observed in practice are described in the Appendix. Table 6.1 summarises these techniques, giving a brief description of each method including:

- indicating whether it elicits values explicitly or implicitly
- how respondents are constrained in expressing their preference and whether or not they are permitted to indicate intensity of preference
- whether respondents have a constrained (forced) choice or an unconstrained choice
- implications of aggregation
- transparency of the technique to users and respondents
- ease of use, especially for respondents
- where relevant, an indication of limits on the applicability of the technique.

The list of techniques described in Table 6.1 is by no means exhaustive. For example, approaches using fuzzy sets, which it is claimed can show a considerable improvement on non-fuzzy approaches, are not covered (Turksen and Willson, 1994).

Table 6.1: Some methods of eliciting preferences

Technique and description	Constraints on respondents	Implications of aggregation	Notes
Single vote Each respondent is given one vote to allocate to their preferred option. Explicit	Respondents forced to give 100% of their 'vote' to preferred option. Constrained choice	If votes are summed, there is inter-respondent equity. Scope for strategic voting.	Transparent, easy to use. However, single winner, first-past-the-post can produce perverse results.
Multiple vote Each respondent given k votes to allocate one each to their k preferred options. Explicit	Respondents forced to give equal $100/k\%$ of vote to each of k options. Constrained	If votes summed, there is inter-respondent equity. Potential for strategic voting.	Transparent, easy to use. If respondents forced to use all their votes, block voting by a group can dominate. (Multiple vote is special case of budget pie.)
Ranking Each respondent asked to rank all or top k options in order of preference. Explicit	Respondents able to indicate order but unable to express intensity of preference. Equal intervals and a fixed intensity of preference are implied if rank positions are treated as cardinal scores. Constrained	Inter-respondent equity. If rank positions are treated as cardinal scores and summed (e.g. Borda count) Arrow's Condition 3 *independence of irrelevant alternatives* can be violated.	Transparent. Easy to use but aggregation can be misleading. (If only first choices are used in aggregation, this method becomes single vote.)
Budget pie (Clark, 1974) (constant sum measurement; point voting system) Each respondent given fixed 'budget' of points/tokens (often 100) or money to allocate between options in any amounts they choose. Explicit	Allows respondents to indicate relative intensity of preference. Constrained	If 'points' summed, inter-respondent equity. Aggregation relatively unproblematic. Little scope for strategic voting.	Transparent. Easy to use (although that is disputed). Can be problems of scale when using money so points or tokens preferred. 'Budget' must contain sufficient points/tokens to permit discrimination in allocation. Useful when options in competition but not mutually exclusive.

Technique and description	Constraints on respondents	Implications of aggregation	Notes
Scoring/rating Each respondent asked to give score/mark/ rating to each option (usually within a defined range). Explicit	Allows respondents to indicate intensity of preference/value. Unconstrained	Inter-respondent inequity if scores given to each option summed (unless each individual's scores are first normalised).	Transparent. Respondents can find the task difficult. Useful when options are not in competition.
Scaling: Likert Scale For each option respondents asked to select position on 'scale' with between five or more 'points'. 'Points' on the scale are usually categories (e.g. strongly agree to strongly disagree). Explicit	Within restrictions of 'scale', allows respondents to indicate intensity of preference. Equal intervals and fixed intensity of preference are imposed if scale 'points' or categories are subsequently converted into scores. Unconstrained	Inter-respondent inequity if 'scores' for each option summed. Frequency counts of respondents' choices of category of scale 'point' for each item/question are relatively unproblematic.	Relatively easy to use, but requires careful design. The imposition of numerical 'scores' on categories can prove misleading.
Scaling: visual analogue scale (VAS) Respondents indicate value of each option on a visual scale (usually marked 0–10 or 0–100). The scale is sometimes presented in a 'thermometer' format. Explicit	Allows respondents to indicate intensity of preference. Unconstrained	Inter-respondent inequity if scores summed for each item (unless each individual's scores first normalised).	Transparent. Easy to use. Useful where options not in competition.
Delphi-type methods Respondents individually value each option, estimate date by which an event will occur, or estimate probability of event occurring. Explicit	Where relevant, permits respondents to indicate intensity of preference. Unconstrained	Results usually presented in histogram format showing responses of every individual for each item.	Transparent. Method of presentation avoids aggregation problems. However, there is often an attempt to achieve consensus through successive rounds.

Technique and description	Constraints on respondents	Implications of aggregation	Notes
Simple paired comparison (dominance preference; discrete choice) Respondents state preference between each pair of options. Frequently used within more complex approaches. Explicit	Respondents unable to indicate intensity of preference. Constrained	If options ranked for each individual, effect is same as ranking above. If aggregated for each pair of options, the voting paradox may prove a problem. Inter-respondent equity.	Relatively transparent. Easy to use but a very large number of comparisons are required if there are more than a few options.
Weighted paired comparison (ratio-scale preference) Respondents state degree of preference between each pair of options. Needs complex transformation (such as that used with AHP) to obtain values. Implicit	Allows respondents to indicate intensity of preference. Unconstrained	Inter-respondent inequity if resulting values for each option summed unless first normalised.	Not very transparent. Very large number of comparisons required if there are more than a very few options.
Constant sum paired comparison Respondents given budget of money or points to allocate between two options. Explicit	Allows respondents to indicate intensity of preference. Constrained.	Inter-respondent equity. Aggregation by summing allocation for each option is relatively unproblematic.	Two-option variant of budget pie. Claimed easier to use (Hauser and Shugan, 1980). Large number of comparisons if more than a few options. Variants of this method limit the set of permitted responses.
Scaled paired comparison Respondents indicate, on a scale, their relative preference between two options. Option values then computed by complex methodology (e.g. priority search or conjoint analysis). Implicit	Allows respondents to indicate intensity of preference. Usually constrained	Depends on method of analysis, but probably equity between respondents.	Not transparent but easy to use for respondents. With some methods of converting to option values, this method is a special case of constant sum paired comparison.

Technique and description	Constraints on respondents	Implications of aggregation	Notes
AHP (analytical hierarchy process) (Saaty, 1977, 1997) Multistage method using weighted paired comparison with limited range of weights. Preferences entered into matrix and converted mathematically into values using eigenvectors. Implicit	Allows respondents to indicate intensity of preference. Initially unconstrained	Aggregation issues not fully addressed. Values are usually normalised.	Not very transparent. Can involve a large number of comparisons. Very widely used, with a large OR and management science literature. Usually used within a decision hierarchy. Range of software available.
Conjoint analysis Options, each with different mix of values of the relevant attributes, presented to respondents, often in pairs. Respondents choose between pair (discrete choice) or rank or rate options. Multiple regression analysis of choices to determine coefficients or weights for each attribute. Implicit	Respondents unable to indicate intensity of preference with simple paired comparison or ranking. However, weighted or scaled paired comparison or rating sometimes used. Constrained	Equity between respondents. Aggregation implicit in multiple regression to obtain coefficients for attributes.	Not transparent. Claimed to be grounded in expected utility theory. The very large number of options possible for every combination of attribute values is usually reduced to make the number of comparisons viable.
Measure of value (based on Churchman and Ackoff, 1954) Respondents first rank options or attributes, then are offered a series of simple paired comparisons between single higher valued options and combination of lower valued options. Option values assigned in accordance with choices. Implicit	Combinations effectively permit respondents to indicate intensity of preference. Unconstrained	If individuals' values summed, interrespondent inequity unless values normalised. Group 'voting' on each decision choice can lead to voting paradox problems.	Not very transparent. Easy to use but needs respondent/researcher (or computer) interaction. Little evidence of recent use.

Technique and description	Constraints on respondents	Implications of aggregation	Notes
Time trade-off Respondents select between higher state of health for shorter period or lower state of health for longer period; or asked how much time they are prepared to lose from life to move from lower state of health to perfect health. Responses converted into values for each health state. Somewhat explicit	Allows respondents to indicate intensity of preference. Constrained	Usually aggregation carried out by computing mean responses. Inter-respondent equity.	Fairly transparent. Evidence of respondent reluctance to trade even small amounts of life for perfect health.
Standard gamble Respondents determine p (probability at which they are indifferent) in gamble between certainty of state of health S and $(1-p)$ probability of perfect health with p probability of death. Value of health state S relative to perfect health and death is determined from the value of p. Implicit	Allows respondents to indicate intensity of preference. Constrained	Usually aggregation by computing mean values. Inter-respondent equity.	Not very transparent. Evidence that respondents have difficulty dealing with probability. Evidence of reluctance to accept even a small risk of death. Widely used by economists in many contexts.
Willingness to pay (WTP) Respondents asked how much they would be willing to pay for product/service or how much more they would pay for some change in service. Explicit?	Allows respondents to indicate relative intensity of preference but affected by disposable income. Effectively unconstrained	Aggregation usually by addition or calculation of means. Inter-respondent equity compromised by differential 'purchasing power' and fact that decisions are effectively unconstrained. Some attempts have been made to weight responses according to income (Donaldson, 1995).	Fairly transparent. Cannot deal with joint products. When applied to public health services, problems of differential purchasing power would appear insuperable. Evidence of resistance from respondents when asked WTP in connection with 'free' health services.

Technique and description	Constraints on respondents	Implications of aggregation	Notes
Qualitative discriminant process (Bryson et al.,1994) Uses VRN (vague real numbers). Respondents assign options to broad categories on each criterion, then to sub-categories within each category and then to sub-subcategories within those. If two or more options still exist in any sub-sub-category, they should be ranked. Partially explicit	Respondents appear to be given some ability to indicate intensity of preference. Constrained to some extent.	In group version, facilitator determines if sufficient degree of consensus. If not, informs decision makers and they repeat individual procedures 'if they feel another round would improve the outcome'. Facilitator generates LP (linear programming) formulation (objective function – minimise difference between 'group' score for each option and score given by each individual).	Does not appear very transparent. Appears to produce group result (i.e. point estimates for each option), but facilitators should 'present each decision maker with his/her vector of scores'. Group version would probably work where reasonable consensus, but not where values very different. Basic (i.e. individual non-group) method may prove useful for eliciting values.
Simple trade-off (compensation or sacrifice) Respondents presented with *status quo* and asked to indicate services for increased expenditure with equivalent number for reduced expenditure. Explicit	Respondents cannot fully indicate intensity of preference. Constrained	Inter-respondent equity. Aggregation normally by summing number indicating reduced expenditure for each item and number indicating increased expenditure for each item.	Transparent and easy to use. Does not easily produce cardinal valuations of options or service changes. The priority evaluator (Hoinville and Courtenay, 1979) is more sophisticated version with similarities to budget pie.
Priority search List of 14–42 services and attributes (mixed) drawn up. Respondents indicate scale preference between limited number of pairs (each attribute/service appears three times). Ranking for each individual service or attribute produced via commercial computer program. Implicit	Allows respondents to indicate intensity of preference. Constrained	Apparently inter-respondent equity. Aggregation by calculating means of rank positions or by deriving 'scores' from the percentage of times that item appears in the top 1/3rd rank positions minus the percentage of times it appears in the bottom 1/3rd rank positions.	Not transparent. Fairly easy for respondents, but large number of comparison choices to make, despite the fact that each option appears only three times. Claimed to be based on personal construct theory (Kelly, 1963) but actual algorithm is commercial secret. Mainly used in local government but some uses in NHS.

Technique and description	Constraints on respondents	Implications of aggregation	Notes
Constrained rating Respondents asked to allocate 'budget' of, say, 4 'very importants' VI, 4 'quite importants' QI and 4 'not impor- tants' NI between 12 options. Scores allo- cated, for example, VI=3 points, QI=2 points, NI=1 point. Explicit?	Allows respondents some limited scope to indicate intensity of preference. (Scoring system forces fixed intensity allocations.) Presentation of ques- tions can appear similar to Likert Scale or to budget pie. Constrained	Inter-respondent equity. 'Scores' summed for each option and often mean 'scores' are computed. Result often presented as overall ranking of options.	Not very transparent. Fairly easy for respon- dents. May mislead respondents because of method of presentation and because conver- sion 'scale' is not usually presented. Users may not under- stand the implications of the technique.
Aggregated scores Respondents score 'performance' of each option on a unique scale for each attribute (e.g. 0–3, 1–5). Option values are calculated by summing scores over all attributes. Explicit	Allows respondents to indicate 'intensity' of 'performance'. Respondents not normally permitted to influence attribute weights (i.e. the maximum permitted scores for each attribute). Effectively unconstrained	Potential inequity between respondents. Values usually summed over all respondents.	Not very transparent. Fairly easy to use, although respondents (and users) may be misled over pre- assigned attribute values/weights. Essentially a two-stage model but the implica- tions of the additive model not always understood by users.

Choice of technique

In selecting or recommending methods for eliciting values, there is a major question of how far it is necessary to be concerned with their theoretical bases. Some claim that it is essential that the technique is grounded in the theory of their own discipline. For instance, most economists would favour only methods involving constrained choices since to economists, 'The concept of value is intimately connected to individual will- ingness to make a sacrifice' (Tideman, 1997, p.226). Some may insist, for example, on psychometric validity. Others may take a far more pragmatic approach.

Whilst acknowledging the theoretical debates, it is suggested for most practical purposes that a pragmatic stance be adopted. Thus, it is suggested, the questions listed in Box 6.3 should be asked of any proposed technique or approach when considering its appropriateness for a particular application. An approach or method which is ideal in one situation may prove totally inappropriate or misleading in another.

Box 6.3:   Questions to be asked of techniques

Appropriateness
- Is the technique appropriate to the problem or issues to which it is to be applied?
- Does it take account of how the problem or issue is likely to be perceived by respondents?
- Are the ways in which respondents are permitted to answer meaningful both to them and to the problem?
- Does the technique seek constrained or unconstrained choices?
- Does the technique permit respondents to indicate intensity of preference?
- How exactly are responses to be interpreted?

Aggregation
- Are the implications of aggregation fully understood by the user?
- Is the aggregation method appropriate to the situation?
- Is any inter-respondent inequity intentional?

Ease of Use and Comprehension
- How easy is the technique for respondents to use?
- How transparent is the technique to the respondents and to users?
- Are its implications generally understood by users?
- Does the technique require (skilled) interviewers or can self-completion methods be used?

The first group of questions relate to the appropriateness or relevance of the technique or approach, both to the overall problem or issue being tackled and to the type of 'options' being presented. For example, if the aim is to obtain general information on values to inform purchasing, asking lay people to rank or allocate sums of money to different treatments for different conditions is unlikely to yield useful information and may encounter respondent resistance.

As discussed earlier, an important consideration is whether or not it is necessary to require respondents to trade off between options. Clearly, if the options are not in competition an 'unconstrained' method would be appropriate. However, even if options are in some sense in competition, it may not be appropriate or useful to force respondents to trade one against another. This was illustrated with the earlier example of a ramp for wheelchair access competing with a play area. To take another case, consider a set of options competing for funding, which include a night-sitting service for the elderly to relieve carers and a neighbourhood walk-in child clinic. If the aim is to determine the relative importance to the community of each service – to determine, say, how many people will be positively affected – it may be more appropriate to ask respondents, using a scale or score, to 'value' the importance to them of each service than to require them to trade off between the services. If the former approach is used, a person who is both a parent of young children and a carer of an elderly person may score both services highly, while a person with no such commitments will score both low. Similarly, if attributes or criteria, such as equity and access, are being valued, an unconstrained approach may be appropriate for eliciting values, even if the resulting values are subsequently normalised. In other cases, the purpose of the exercise may well be to introduce respondents to the concept of trade-off or sacrifice and/or to determine their preference or choice under such conditions. In such cases a constrained method would be indicated. However, if options are mutually exclusive, some methodologies which constrain choices, such as budget pie and its variants, will not work. Box 6.4 suggests some questions which should be asked to ensure an appropriate method is selected, including whether a constrained and/or an unconstrained method is indicated.

Box 6.4:   Questions to be asked of options

- Are the options in competition?
- Are the options mutually exclusive?
- Are the options complementary?
- Are the options inter-related?
- Are the options independent?

In many cases, it is desirable to permit respondents to indicate their intensity of preference. Special care should be taken with methodologies which either implicitly force an intensity of preference to be indicated which may not accord with the respondent's values (e.g. multiple vote) or subsequently impose a specific intensity of preference on the respondent's choices, of which the respondent may not be aware (e.g. the use of rank positions as 'scores' or the assumption of 'equally appearing intervals' for responses on a Likert Scale). However, in some cases, the purpose of the exercise may be to force a choice between two or more options and thus expressions of intensity of preference may be inappropriate.

Methodologies which involve money, such as some variants of budget pie and willingness to pay (WTP), can raise problems. Willingness to pay approaches can encounter problems with respondent resistance or undervaluation where the options for which WTP is being sought are normally provided free. Further, despite some imaginative attempts (Donaldson, 1995), the problem of the influence of respondents' differential purchasing power has not been satisfactorily solved. In addition, willingness to pay might appear at first sight to be the archetypal constrained method involving as it does 'notions of sacrifice'; however, when used to value publicly provided services which are competing within a constrained budget, it effectively offers an unconstrained choice to respondents or at least a choice constrained only by their own personal disposable income, not the public budget.

Budget pie and its two-option variant, constant sum paired comparison, overcome these problems as respondents are allocated a 'budget'. However, the choice of the absolute size of the budget to be allocated may raise problems; should the sums involved be realistic and thus probably outside the normal experience of respondents or should they be token, e.g. £100, and risk seeming trivial? Examination of some applications suggests that budget pie-type methods may work better when respondents are 'given' tokens or points rather than cash. With tokens or points, however, sufficient (often 100) must be allocated to permit respondents enough discrimination in allotting them between options. One study, which allowed a budget of only 15 tokens, reported respondents wishing to cut tokens in half.

The second set of questions in Box 6.3 relate to aggregation. Here, it is important that the researcher/user understands the implications of any aggregation that is carried out and relates them to the context of the problem. In many instances, a method of summarising, rather than aggregating, which demonstrates the range of responses, e.g. the Delphi method of presentation (see Fig. 6.1), may be more appropriate than a method which sums choices or scores across respondents. Simply arguing that societal choices have to be made and proceeding to 'average' diametrically opposite views or values is frequently inappropriate.

A second problem with aggregation is whether respondents are, or should be, given equal weight. Several techniques, e.g. voting and budget pie, give respondents equal weight unless a deliberate choice is made to give unequal weights by giving respondents unequal numbers of votes or unequal budgets. However, aggregation using some methodologies gives respondents unequal weights in a way which may be unintended by the researcher/user, e.g. where respondents have been permitted to allocate unconstrained scores to options or where rank positions have been summed (with or without reversing the 'scores') and some respondents have ranked the whole list of options and others only their top few choices. In some applications, for instance the examples of a night-sitting service versus a child clinic and the ramp versus the play area, allowing some respondents greater 'weight' overall than others might be considered desirable and appropriate. It would, however, seem important not to allow accidental inter-respondent inequity. Normalisation of respondents' scores can be used when inter-respondent equity is required.

The third group of questions relate to ease of use, comprehension and transparency, in respect of both the researcher/user and the respondents. It is important that the researcher/user understands the techniques being used, their implications and, in particular, the way in which final 'scores' are produced and their interpretation. Dangers can especially arise from the use of computer software where it permits users to employ methodologies which they do not fully understand.

From the point of view of respondents, in general it is desirable that the chosen technique is easy to use. However, whether or not techniques need to be, or should be, transparent to respondents – in the sense that they can see how their responses are going to be used and how they contribute to the final scores – will depend on the application. Thus, although transparency may generally be preferred, there may well be cases when lack of transparency is an essential part of the research process but this latter circumstance should not be abused. However, greater understanding of the methodology and its working on the part of respondents might increase the danger of strategic 'voting', mentioned above.

Comparisons of various techniques for valuing and eliciting preferences, mostly drawing on empirical studies, can be found *inter alia* in Bard (1992); Bombardier *et al.* (1982); Brooks and O'Leary (1983); Brown and Jackson (1978); Buede and Maxwell (1995); Camasso and Dick (1993); Carr-Hill (1989); Clark (1976); Deber and Geol (1990); Dodd and Donegan (1995); Hadorn (1991a); Hauser and Shugan (1980); Kind (1988); Millet (1997); Rothermel and Schilling (1984); and Triantaphyllou *et al.* (1994). In addition to discussing methods of eliciting values, the following consider the implications of different methods of aggregation: Dyer and Forman (1992); Jensen (1986); Perez (1994); Perez and Barbra-Romero (1995); and Torrance (1986).

The pragmatic approach to the choice of methodology has some long-standing support. For instance, Huber (1974), demonstrating that under many circumstances different methods of eliciting values, and indeed different formulations of the MAU model, are equally good predictors of clients' preferences, concludes that transparency is important and that acceptability of the model and method to the client should be the major choice criterion. Clark (1974, p.26) suggests that 'One good principle is to utilize instruments only as precise and complex as necessary for the decision at hand', adding that 'the instruments can be no more sensitive than their users'. However, it should not be concluded that it is unimportant which method is chosen. In a small-scale study, comparing a method which permitted expression of intensity of preference (budget pie) with one which did not (multiple vote), Mullen (1983) demonstrated that very different individual and aggregated group values resulted.

CHAPTER SEVEN

Priority-setting approaches in practice

Some approaches to priority setting outside the NHS

As is obvious from the wide range of techniques available and the depth of some of the debates, eliciting preferences and values has a very long history, in some cases many centuries, although much of the earlier work was devoted to elections and voting. Interest in involving the public and eliciting their values has varied over time. For instance, in the US from time to time legislation is passed encouraging or requiring public consultation or involvement. In the UK, there was an upsurge of interest in eliciting public preferences in the 1970s, especially in connection with local authority structure plans. Value elicitation is also used in priority-setting exercises among professionals and within the private sector. Studies illustrating a range of approaches are discussed below.

Studies using multiple approaches and techniques

Hoinville and Courtenay (1979) describe a structure plan survey, carried out in 1972–73, with the aim of measuring the importance to Merseyside residents of 37 environmental problems identified by the project team. This study used three separate measures: (1) rank ordering of problems experienced; (2) a four-point scale rating of the seriousness of each problem as experienced by respondents; (3) a budget pie method, with each respondent having 20 discs to allocate among the first ten problems ranked. Nine different scoring methods were explored before choosing one to calculate an 'improvement score' for each option. However, although the different methods yielded different responses, generally the mean (aggregated) results correlated highly.

In a more recent study, Camasso and Dick (1993) also used a range of value elicitation techniques but at different stages of the exercise rather than as alternatives. The study involved the Essex County New Jersey Advisory Council, which consists of representatives of the general public, service consumers and providers of services, who were charged with needs assessment of target (at-risk) populations and preparing a list of 15 ranked service priorities. In the first stage of the study, three opinion surveys (of informed citizens (265), clients (284) and professionals (140)) were conducted in which respondents were asked to assign a priority to 62 problems/issues facing 18 at-risk/target populations using a five-point scale, ranging from much lower priority to much higher priority. The results were used to produce rankings of the top 20 items for each of the three groups. In the second stage, participants (Advisory Council members divided into small groups) were given two hours to study the data from the survey, social indicator data organised into five major groups (economic well-being, health status, family functioning, crime and education) presented at municipality level and compared with state-wide data, plus *A Dictionary of Standardized Target Problem Definitions*. They were then presented with a problem cluster tree, the base branches of which (economic opportunity issues, health issues, education issues, family/child development issues, crime and delinquency issues) – the principal interest areas – were derived from the groups employed in the indicator analysis. Participants were asked to divide 100 points between the five 'principal interest areas' according to their view of how critical and important they were. Participants were then asked, drawing on all the information they had been provided with, to enter up to six subbranches against each of the five 'principal interest areas' and then asked to allocate a total of five points among the six subbranches within each 'principal interest area' (it is not clear whether these five points could be allocated in 'units' of less than 1). In the third stage, weights were computed for each subbranch for each participant by multiplying the points allocated to a subbranch within its 'principal interest area' by the points allocated to that 'principal interest area'. In the fourth stage, each participant was asked to score each of 30 services against each subbranch on a 1–100 scale (1=meet problem completely, 100 = not meet problem at all) – the service impact rating. In stage five, a score for each service was computed by multiplying the subbranch weight by the appropriate service impact rating, the resulting scores being averaged over the 51 participants. The 15 services with the highest mean service scores were ranked according to those scores and presented to the decision makers.

Another study using a variety of value-eliciting techniques, this time for public participation in community planning in a small town, is described by Sancar (1993). One hundred and fifty individuals were identified covering 13 interest or stakeholder groups. They were sent a questionnaire "to sample opinions on various social, economic and physical issues", plus an invitation (accepted by 43) to attend a series of workshops. The first workshop, which aimed 'to develop a mission statement, identify individual attitudes about planning and obtain an initial account of the participants' perceptions and points of view', used a modified 'root definition' technique developed by Checkland. In the second workshop, which dealt with issues in planning relating to resources and problems, participants were divided into groups of four, first drawing up lists individually, then debating them in the groups and eventually combining them for the whole workshop. To avoid problems associated with 'conventional' ranking of issues, in particular the elimination of minority views, in the third workshop participants analysed the relationships between issues in two interaction matrices containing problems and opportunities, apparently using a cross-impact approach. A computer program, using interpretive structural modelling, generated network diagrams that represented the cumulative thinking of all the groups. In the fourth workshop the network diagrams were presented to participants, who were asked to identify major issues and questions to be asked for future development. The questions were voted on and ranked according to the number of votes received.

A 'Policy Delphi' was then conducted in front of an audience of participants, with a panel of six experts considering three scenarios which had been identified in advance. The experts were asked to estimate how the way of life (in terms of levels of employment and occupation, population and housing, household income and retail sales) would change under each scenario. After each estimate, the experts shared their valuations and discussed differences of opinion.

Drawing on the results of the workshops and the Policy Delphi, the project team formulated design proposals for each of three future scenarios for each of six sites within the city. These were evaluated by the participants in the final workshop, after which the community design proposals were displayed at three prominent places in the city for three weeks. Citizens viewing the exhibits were asked which site interested them most and were then requested to evaluate, through a series of questions, the three options for that site. In addition to being asked to rate how pleasant, stimulating and attractive the design proposals were, respondents were asked to specify their overall preference for each scenario by distributing 100 points. An interesting finding was that the general public liked the proposals more than the participants in the workshops.

Budget pie and related approaches

All three of the above applications employed the budget pie method alongside other techniques. There are many other applications of the budget pie method, alone and in combination with other techniques. Clark (1974) cites a range of applications including within the police and other public services, using a variety of different presentations to respondents, including pie slices, $ pegs and poker chips. There are many variants of the budget pie method. In a recent health service application in the US, Garland (1992) describes its use in Oregon where the commissioners each distributed 100 points among three broad value attributes. In a variant, Strauss and Hughes (1976) describe a study, involving a random sample of 1000 residents of North Carolina, which used a budget pie in the form of 15 coupons, which could be allocated to expenditure increases and/or tax reductions.

The number of 'points' allocated to respondents may be significant, over and above considerations of allowing enough points to permit sufficiently fine distinctions whilst not overwhelming respondents, mentioned in Chapters Four and Six. Hoinville and Courtenay (1979) describe an exercise in which the number of points available was successively reduced. Respondents, however, did not reduce their allocation to each option/aspect proportionately. Some aspects retained all or most of their allocation, thus increasing their share of the 'pie'. However, it is not clear whether this effect was the result of asking respondents to repeat their allocations with successively fewer points (i.e. effectively moving from their initial allocation) or the result of the absolute number of points permitted at each stage.

Unless there is a justified reason for allowing inequity, the budget pie method is usually operated with an equal number of points for each respondent. However, Hoinville and Courtenay (1979) cite studies of housing conditions and environment, conducted in Runcorn and in Milton Keynes, which allowed tenants to 'buy' additional points to add to their budget pie, provided they said they were prepared to take an increase in rent. Returning to the Merseyside study (described above), Hoinville and Courtenay suggest that the equal 'disc' allocation has limitations in that a person with one problem can allocate all 20 discs to it, whilst a person with five problems has to share the 20 discs between all five. They suggest that this could be overcome by giving more discs to those with more problems or by subsequently weighting their score. However, any such 'weighting' must be used with caution as it would appear to negate many of the stated advantages of the budget pie.

The simple trade-off (compensation or sacrifice) method was used in a South York Structure Plan survey (Courtenay and Field, 1975). Ten local facilities or environmental aspects were listed and, for each one, respondents were asked to indicate (by moving discs from the central 'present position') whether they would accept a lower standard, would choose the present situation or wanted improvement. Initially this was posed without constraints. The exercise was then repeated but respondents had to 'compensate' every aspect they chose for improvement with the 'sacrifice' of a lowered standard for another aspect. Unsurprisingly, far fewer improvements were sought and far more 'sacrifices' were offered with the constrained method.

Hoinville and Courtenay (1979) describe a more sophisticated version of this approach – the priority evaluator – which is related to the budget pie. Respondents first identify their current position (e.g. their present housing and environmental situation) on separate scales for each attribute. The scores corresponding to their current position are summed to give a total score or 'budget', which respondents can then reallocate across the attribute scales. Thus to keep within the 'budget', improvements must be compensated for by 'dis-improvements'. Experience shows that respondents can easily cope with up to ten scales in one exercise. Since respondents' individual starting positions may affect their subsequent 'scoring', strictly analysis should compare respondents starting in the same/similar positions. Further, it is noted that respondents who start off in a poor position continue to be disadvantaged, as they have fewer points to 'play' with. To overcome this problem, one suggestion is that everyone could be given the same points to begin with (which would effectively be a standard budget pie); another suggestion is that there should be a set minimum to the number of points allocated to any respondent.

Ranking

Ranking, often accompanied by the calculation of mean rank positions, is probably the most common technique and appears in many studies in many different fields. Accompanying discussion exhibits varying degrees of comprehension of the implications of this deceptively simple approach. Several instances of ranking were observed in the examples of multiple approaches discussed above.

Jefferson and Demicheli (1995) describe a priority setting exercise relating to British Forces Germany Health Services, which are being subjected to market testing. An anonymous two-page questionnaire, asking respondents to rank (1–10) ten services (eight given and two written-in 'other') and to rank (1–6) six characteristics of health services (five given and one written-in 'other'), was distributed by various methods, requesting that one be completed per household. The services and characteristics given had been chosen from discussions by focus groups. The results from the questionnaire are presented as combined rank position and in the form of diagrams showing 'spatial distribution' using median, 25th and 75th percentiles for ranks given to each service/characteristic. The exercise then moved on to a priority-setting panel discussion, involving a lay panel and a healthcare workers panel. The lay panel members were asked to read BAOR Report of Public Health 1992–93 and the healthcare workers panel the preliminary findings of the priority rating questionnaires. Nominal group techniques and the Delphi technique, adapted 'to fit a military setting', were used. Consensus was achieved by two rounds, each involving first 'a self-generated list of services and then a priority voting' (method not specified but appears to be ranking). 'Mean priority rating scores' (mean rank positions?) for each service for each panel separately and combined are presented. Final rankings of the services are based on these 'mean priority rating scores'.

Scaling/rating

The use of scaling and rating in value elicitation is also very common. However, not only do such scales have to be designed and presented with care, there are risks of scale and order effects. Knox (1977), reporting a large national survey scoring importance of life domains each on an 11-point ladder scale, found the results skewed towards the top end of the scale. Hoinville and Courtenay (1979) describe a method of presenting a scale with 'opposite' statements at each end, with respondents being asked to indicate their own position on the scale. 'Order' effects were tested for by reversing the position of the two statements for half the respondents. The results revealed a marked 'order' effect with respondents tending to endorse the right-hand box.

Measure of Value

Although Huber (1974, 1975) refers to it as the 'well known' Measure of Value, this technique does not appear to have been widely used in recent years. Churchman and Ackoff (1954) describe the application of Measure of Value to evaluating five-year objectives of an American corporation and also cite its use in assigning weights to criteria used in the selection of potential public housing sites. In another US example, Stimson (1971) describes the use of Measure of Value in health agency decision making.

Analytical hierarchy process (AHP)

Since the publication of the first article (Saaty, 1977) AHP has been widely used, especially in the US but also in the the UK and other European countries. Many applications are found within industry and private sector organisations but AHP has also been used within the public sector. For instance, among many other applications, Rabinowitz (1992) describes the application of AHP to resource allocation decisions in urban renewal projects and resource allocation for human resources development plans. Greenberg and Nunamaker (1994) describe a problem of multicriteria budgetary allocation in public sector organisation. A linear model is used with the objective to maximise $\Sigma x_j.c_{jk}$ (where x = total dollars allocated to department j and c_{jk} = the jth department's marginal contribution per dollar to objective k). AHP was used to determine the decision makers' assessment of the relative contribution weights w_{jk}, which were scaled to yield c_{jk}. Algie et al. (1983) used priority scaling, a method very similar to AHP, to assist in determining priorities within a social services department faced with financial cuts. In a series of studies, Dolan and others have used AHP to involve patients in medical decision making. Dolan and Bordley (1993) describe the (potential) use of AHP to assist patients in choosing between four different treatment regimes to reduce the risk of getting a particular (non-specified) disease. Dolan and Bordley (1994) go on to discuss its (potential) use in determining whether or not to administer isoniazid prophylaxis to individuals with positive TB tests, but with no clinical symptoms of TB. Dolan (1995) used 20 volunteers to evaluate the use of AHP in making decisions about different screening programmes for cancer of the colon. He concluded (p.79) that 'the results indicate that AHP-based decision-making aids are likely to be acceptable to and within the capabilities of many patients ...'.

Although the AHP method usually requires direct interaction between the decision makers and the facilitator or computer program, Choi et al. (1994) describe an application using self-completion questionnaires in the choice of a city to become the new provincial capital. A series of pairwise questions were sent to 87 academics (apparently considered to be a relatively objective group) and 37 response sheets were returned. The responses were analysed using the 'Expert Choice' AHP computer package.

However, despite its widespread use over many years, the 1–9 (Saaty) scale used in AHP has remained controversial. Bard (1992) compared AHP with multi-attribute utility theory (MAUT) in a problem involving the selection of rough terrain cargo handlers for the US Army. Five programme managers and engineers evaluated three alternatives according to four criteria. Individual results were aggregated using arithmetic and geometric means. Apart from the restrictions of the 1–9 scale, the participants generally found AHP easier and less time consuming to use. In particular, in the MAUT analysis participants found difficulty with the standard gamble, especially when working with very low probabilities. Dodd and Donegan (1995), in a theoretical article comparing prioritisation techniques, discuss the potential shortcomings of the AHP (Saaty) 1–9 scale. Some problems seem to centre round the fact that Saaty phrases are soft but his methodology requires hard ratios. Like several other commentators, they also focus on the problems and interpretation of the reciprocal of the 1–9 scale. Triantaphyllou *et al.* (1994), noting recent suggestions that the original Saaty scale may cause severe inconsistencies in many decision-making problems and that exponential scales seem to be more natural for humans in decision making, use two criteria to evaluate 78 different scales. However, no single scale outperforms all others, but a few are efficient under certain conditions.

Valuing of health status indices, QALYs, etc.

Values are involved in the construction of health status indices, which can be used in economic appraisal and priority setting in the form of QALYs or similar measures. In addition to the never-ending debate about whose values should be used, there is widespread debate on the methodologies used for eliciting and aggregating values. The resulting scales can prove important in practice. For example, the apparently counter-intuitive rankings initially produced using the Quality of Well-being (QWB) Scale in the Oregon exercise were attributed by Nord (1993) to the unfounded assumption that QWB values have cardinal properties, whilst at the same time the methods used for eliciting values resulted in insufficient compression of values at the top end of the scale. Among many contributions to the debate, Torrance (1986) and Torrance and Feeney (1989) discuss and compare methods of utility measurement, including rating scale (using different health states for the same duration), standard gamble, time trade-off and multi-attribute utility theory, also debating at length the problems of interpersonal aggregation. Nord (1990), commenting on the argument that utility weights valuing health states are meaningless, argues that we 'should be careful to distinguish between two different ways of establishing utility weights' – rating scales and trade-off techniques. He argues that there is a problem with a 0–100 rating scale because few respondents use numerical scales in everyday situations when thinking of or expressing quality of life. On the other hand, although trade-off techniques (time trade-off [as described in Chapter Six and the Appendix] or choosing between spending £1 million curing ten type A patients or spending £1 million curing 100 type B patients) are not easy, 'many people are faced with precisely this kind of question in real life ... In this sense trade-off questions seem quite meaningful'. Thus, although the validity of QALYs is debatable, Nord claims that it is wrong to claim that numerical valuations of health states are meaningless, provided they are obtained by trade-off methods.

Some approaches to priority setting within the NHS

Priority-setting exercises have been carried out within the NHS for a long time. For example, Dickinson (1979) described the use of Measure of Value by the Hereford Health District Planning Team to attach values (or priority weights) to plan proposals before forwarding them to the area health authority. However, as noted above, within the new NHS there is increasing interest in priority setting, including exercises involving the public, with the stated intention of informing the purchasing plans of health authorities. Of particular headline interest are instances of health authorities refusing completely to purchase a particular service.

However, despite the sometimes rather 'macho' debate, there is evidence that few health authorities have completely excluded purchasing particular forms of treatment. Klein and Redmayne (1992), in their survey, found only 12 purchasers out of 114 had decided to discontinue purchasing specific services. Where services/treatment are excluded they are usually fairly peripheral and relatively easy targets, e.g. *in vitro* fertilisation (IVF), stripping of varicose veins, tattoo removal, cosmetic surgery and gender reassignment (Redmayne, 1992; Redmayne and Klein, 1993). Less 'macho' forms of rationing take the form of limiting the number of treatments purchased and agreeing treatment protocols with providers.

A survey of all health authorities within the UK was conducted by the authors in 1994–95, seeking information about projects and exercises involving the public in priority setting. The aim of this survey was specifically to obtain examples of techniques used and of the impact of such exercises on purchasing/priority setting; thus it was not the aim of the survey to determine the extent of consumer involvement. The majority of information was obtained in response to a letter and pro forma sent to directors of public health in all the then health authorities in the UK. Additional information was obtained by phone, letter and/or visit. Details of the studies were entered on to a database, which has since been interrogated by a number of researchers from the NHS and elsewhere.

Of the 179 projects reported in this survey, only a very few sought priorities between whole services and treatments and those that did largely responded to the question asking what influence the project had had on purchasing decisions or priorities by replying simply that the values elicited from the public 'were taken into account'.

Several respondents commented on the value gained from the process of carrying out the exercise, which was independent of any results actually obtained.

Where exercises had sought to obtain the views of the public on, say, the choice between two treatments or between the young and the old, many reported resistance to participating in these more 'macho' priority-setting exercises. A number of respondents either felt that such decisions should be left to professionals, usually doctors, or that rationing and priority setting were a cover for cuts resulting from government underfunding of the health service and they wanted no part of it. Indeed, a survey by Richardson *et al.* (1992) found ambivalent responses from the public about who should make priority-setting decisions and Heginbotham (1993, p.147) reported a survey which showed that only 22% of 'general public' respondents answered that the general public should 'make decisions on which treatment takes a higher priority'.

A large number of the projects reported in our survey sought views on attributes of service delivery, such as geographical location (and resultant access issues), other access issues such as facility opening times and special transport, location of treatment and facilities (e.g. hospital versus community), type of treatment and a range of quality issues. Generally, there appears to be far less public resistance to responding in these areas and there was often a far more direct link with purchasing plans and policy making.

Some respondents discussed the public's lack of knowledge of the structure and organisation of the NHS – in particular the 1991 NHS changes – suggesting that the public cannot usefully contribute to healthcare priority setting until they are educated about NHS structure and financing and understand the roles, responsibilities and relationships of the various bodies within it.

Engaging the public

Priority-setting exercises described in the literature and reported in our survey use a wide range of approaches to involve the public; indeed, examples of almost every approach discussed in Chapter Five are found. However, as the objective of the survey was not to produce a comprehensive picture but to identify interesting and useful examples of priority-setting methodology, the figures and percentages presented here should be treated with caution and taken as illustrative only.

Surveys

Over 40% of projects reported in the survey of health authorities used questionnaire surveys, in one form or another.

The survey approach adopted by the Eastern Surrey Health Commission (MacDonald, 1994) represents a classic example of the difficulty of moving to precision in outcome decisions even when surveys are well conducted. A postal questionnaire was sent to 2500 residents selected at random from the electoral register and a 63%

response rate was achieved. The questions included willingness to travel for treatment to save money for the HA; what travel time respondents consider reasonable for different treatments; and what travel they would be willing to undertake to get better facilities; as well as a request to select four possible service developments for reinvestment from a list of nine. The answers were presented as the percentage ticking that service/aspect.

Although participants were uneasy about making choices and were not totally convinced that the exercise was not simply about cost savings rather than reinvestment, nonetheless priorities were indicated. However, priority was given to fairly common conditions on the basis of the health experience of their age group. It is therefore important for health authorities to take into account views such as these but this is still a significant step away from making a specific and firm decision about a set of priorities.

A public consultation exercise by Gwynedd Community Health Councils (1994) is a typical example of an initiative at a relatively early stage of public participation. The aims of this work were to: (a) introduce the concept of participation in planning and developing a local health strategy; (b) use the information gathered to influence the commissioning of health services. The approach utilised a questionnaire administered in an interview format allowing for additional open comments. Respondents were asked detailed questions on 11 possible but expensive service developments. These were followed by a prioritisation question in which respondents were asked to score each development on a five-point scale (5=absolutely urgent and essential within one year; 4=essential within two years; 3=desirable within three years; 2=desirable within four years; 1=not required).

The sample was never intended to be truly representative of the population of Gwynedd (243 800), since it employed opportunistic rather than random sampling, with the 619 returns being obtained from users of health establishments or individuals who expressed an interest. Perhaps because of this selection process, a very large percentage of respondents had previous awareness of health services they were asked to consider. Whilst people in this sample were happy to offer views on their experience of a service, the prioritisation on the 11 expensive services proved a much more difficult task. A typical comment was that all the services were important and it was too difficult to choose between them on the five-point scale. Some 85% of respondents did undertake the prioritisation task but many allocated equal priority to all services. Palliative care and pain relief service emerged as slightly higher priorities than other services but it was quite marginal.

The authors of the report noted the very high time commitment such processes demand, but perhaps of more general interest is the particular difficulty of respondents who did not have any knowledge of a particular service. Finally, the interview process did produce an extremely large number of individual statements, e.g. we need more centres to cut out travelling or more beds are needed to meet the need for occasional care. Whilst such statements are interesting and provide some insight into the public's thinking, the question of the representativeness of such material is clearly illustrated.

Sandwell Health Authority commissioned Gallup to conduct a survey amongst residents to assess their views on some proposed improvements in local health services over the two years from April 1994 to March 1995 and to rank them. This study combined qualitative and quantitative methods since prior to the interview survey, involving 801 interviews with members of the public selected by stratified random sampling, Gallup conducted three discussion groups. The interviews used a part-coded structured questionnaire mainly concerned with satisfaction with the health service. However, in one two-part question, respondents were to indicate the importance of 14 items on a four-point scale (very important; fairly important; not very important; not at all important) and then asked, 'If money was limited, which two [of the 14] do you think would be most important to you and your family?'.

However, despite the fact that the problem of representativeness frequently associated with qualitative methods can, in theory, be overcome with the more quantitative large-scale survey approach, very low response rates may cause problems. North Staffordshire Health Authority employed a short questionnaire asking respondents to indicate the issues, problems or developments in relation to the health services in the district which they would most like to see considered. Three large spaces were given for responses. The questionnaire was distributed to 36 000 people via the authority's free newspaper, which represented one-sixth of the total distribution. Waiting time for first outpatient appointment and waiting time for operation emerged as key issues, but the response rate overall (216 replies, 0.6%) was extremely low.

Clearly, when engaging the public in priority-setting exercises there is a need to ensure that both adequate background information and a willingness to undertake such a task are in existence.

Meetings

Forty-five (25%) of the 179 projects involved meetings, 27 of which were described as public meetings. Most of the remainder were meetings with consumer and voluntary groups, user groups and/or locality meetings. Attendance at public meetings appears to be affected by the presence of contentious local issues. For instance, Orkney Health Board reported that the three meetings they held to seek views of the public on the Health Board strategy attracted a lot of interest because of fears over the future on long-stay beds. Worcester Health Authority, however, found public meetings not effective and reported that attendance by HA representatives at existing meetings of public groups, clubs and organisations had proved more effective. Wakefield Healthcare established a panel of speakers to go out to talk to local groups and, in another case, a health authority invited local groups to organise a public meeting, with the authority providing speakers and meeting other costs.

Focus groups and panels

Focus groups were also popular, with 56 (31%) of the 179 projects using them. These took a variety of forms, some dealing with general health services issues, such as considering a health authority's plans, and some concentrating on a specific service, user group or issue of local concern. In a number of cases, outside organisations were employed to facilitate such groups.

Southern Derbyshire Health Authority and others (SMSR, 1994) employed focus groups in a public consultation day, adopting a mainly qualitative approach to the task of seeking the public's opinions of the proposals in the HA's five-year plan. A total of seven focus groups (46 participants in all) spent the day in discussion examining the proposals. The output from each group was compiled by a facilitator and at the end of the day each person was asked to complete a short questionnaire to rate the various service items. The groups were also asked to allocate a notional budget of £100 to the competing priorities. A number of the individuals and groups found this task too complicated. At the end of the day, a short questionnaire containing statements was distributed, asking respondents to indicate their agreement/disagreement with the statement on a five-point scale.

The project produced a lot of interesting material (as qualitative approaches tend to) and the authority was certainly in a position to take such views into its decision making. However, as with qualitative studies again, the scope for generalising from the views of the 46 participants (although carefully selected) is limited. Once again, the issue of precisely why the public is being consulted is paramount.

In order to ensure that focus group participants are better informed, Bowie *et al.* (1995) report using an approach similar to that reported by Hoinville and Courtenay (1979). Eight focus groups, each with 12 members, were established, each group meeting three times a year. At each meeting groups are given a real issue to discuss, for which they are given an information briefing. Focus group members are selected by quota sampling techniques and each member has a tenure of one year; thus four members of each group are replaced at each meeting. West Yorkshire Health Authority, in conjunction with the local metropolitan council, report establishing panels of people (the Kirklees Panel has 1018 members, for example), who can be surveyed periodically. Gwent Health Commission, also working in conjunction with local authorities, have been piloting 'health panels', consisting of a representative cross-section of local people (three per 1000) willing to complete questionnaires. In a project called REACT, Argyll and Clyde Health Board are experimenting with a 'panel' of local residents over 15 years old, currently self-selected, all or some section of whom (in line with the areas under research) are sampled for surveys using self-completion questionnaires.

In a slightly different use of panels, the Isle of Wight Health Commission established a panel of enquiry to consider and advise the commission on the need for an island-based medium-stay low-secure unit for those with mental illness and challenging behaviour. The panel took evidence from national and local experts, local voluntary and user groups; members of the public were invited to ask questions and to express views and preferences. According to the informant for the commission, the panel proved to be a very good mechanism for enabling the community to make informed decisions; the public who attended appreciated being involved in the decision-making process and the opportunity to influence service provision; the purchaser and provider representatives found the process challenging, in particular the need to justify intentions. However, it was very time consuming

Rapid appraisal

The approach, which is being used increasingly in the NHS, was reported in nine projects in our survey of health authorities.

Murray *et al.* (1994) describe its use on an Edinburgh estate. Semistructured interviews of 'key' local people, plus 17 local residents, were carried out; the health questions largely asked about what services they used, what was best about them and in what way they could be improved. Respondents were also asked what they thought were the worst health problems in the area and what change they would like to make to the area.

As mentioned in Chapter Five, Ong *et al.* (1991) describe a rapid appraisal carried out in South Sefton designed to help researchers 'define more precisely the nature and magnitude of felt needs'. Subteams of researchers interviewed 'those who would know about the community' – professionals, community leaders and corner shopkeepers. From these interviews, priority areas and issues within them were identified, which were returned to 'the community' for ranking in priority order.

Barking and Havering HA (Singleton, 1994) used the methodology with 30 local health-related professionals and community leaders with the objective of ascertaining the health needs in a defined locality and developing an action plan to address those needs with an emphasis on *Health of the Nation* areas. Although the technique does not in itself produce quantitative data, it was extended to do so in this context. The initial appraisal interviews sought to 'raise health issues'. These issues were placed in groups. From lists of the issues thus raised, respondents were asked to rank the top five from each group list and rank the top ten from all lists. The final list was based on the number of times an item appeared in the top ten. A weighting score was also calculated by using reverse rank positions and summing, in order to indicate strength of feeling. The top three issues to emerge were unemployment, housing and ambulance services. It is not unusual with rapid appraisal to identify such broad all-encompassing categories. The contribution of the various agencies to tackling such issues represented the next stage of the process. In the project conducted here, focus groups were used to feed back the results and a follow-up 'walk-about' survey conducted to assess progress in the various areas.

The relative speed of rapid appraisal must be considered in the light of the intended purpose. If it is more precise priority setting for specific services with a measure of representativeness then rapid appraisal may not be appropriate.

Eliciting values and prioritisation techniques

One-fifth (36) of the projects reported in our survey gave details of the use of one or more explicit valuing or prioritisation techniques. Some of those approaches and techniques, together with examples reported in the published literature, are discussed below.

Ranking

Ranking is by far the most frequently used method (occurring in at least 23 of the 36 projects), both for services/treatments and for attributes of health services. Indeed, so ubiquitous is ranking that the term was used even where some form of rating scale was employed. A majority of studies which used ranking aggregated responses by calculating the mean of the rank positions. However, rankings were also aggregated by presenting the number and/or percentage of first places each option received (equivalent to single vote) and the number and/or percentage of top three places each option received (equivalent to multiple vote).

An interesting example of the use of ranking is given by North West Lancashire Health Authority. The objective was to rank 60 items of healthcare and health authority activity in order of importance. However, since dealing with 60 items in a single exercise would be a virtually impossible psychological task, each questionnaire used in the postal survey of the general public contained a randomly selected list of ten of the 60 items. As an additional feature, in order to test different methodologies, two different versions of the questionnaire were used. Both asked respondents to 'imagine that we have to move money from low need services into high need services'. The first version then asked respondents to place the ten items in rank order (1–10); the second asked respondents to indicate, for each of the ten services, whether they were 'very high need', 'high need', 'low need' or 'very low need'.

The results obtained from the ranking on the sets of ten were combined, producing a rank ordering of the 60 items. Interestingly, 'Ambulances arriving within 10 minutes of 999 call' was first, followed by cancer scans, kidney dialysis and heart bypass operations. There seems to be a technological preference emerging which is not atypical of public judgements.

Single/multiple vote

Versions of the single or multiple vote were used in a variety of formats. In an example of multiple vote, one authority reported widespread distribution of a detailed leaflet outlining 24 possible health initiatives, inviting members of the public to indicate which three they thought most important. Another example of multiple vote occurred in the postal survey conducted for Eastern Surrey Health Commission, mentioned above, where respondents were asked to select the four most important service developments from a list of nine and to tick four aspects of services from a list of ten. The same authority, in another postal survey, used a variant of the multiple vote where respondents were asked to select the three most important and the three least important services in terms of NHS priorities. In a project which employed the single-vote method, respondents to a postal survey were asked which one of five (fairly broad) options they would select if all new money had to go to only one area.

In a postal survey which aimed to identify GP opinions/preferences for service development and to assist with the Board's purchasing process, Dumfries and Galloway Health Board (1994) presented respondents with a list of 45 services. They were asked to give two ticks to a single top priority for service development (single vote) and one tick each to the next four priorities (multiple vote). The results were presented in two tables: one presented the top priorities only (i.e. those services given two ticks), the other gave the overall priorities (i.e. all the services given either one or two ticks). A set of priorities were identified (orthopaedics, physiotherapy, outpatients, clinical psychology, physiotherapy, domiciliary); these are relatively unusual in the total context of priority setting and may well represent a clear concern from one health agent (GPs) about the provision of specific services in a particular local context. It also serves as a note of caution to those who seek to use the views of GPs as a proxy for those of their patients or the general public. As the authority commented, such a priority list is probably best used as a guide to further investigation of these services and how provision might be improved. They also comment that an extension of the process to other populations would be interesting and, of course, potentially problematic if alternative sets of priorities were identified.

Scaling/rating

Scaling and rating appeared in at least 13 projects as well as appearing frequently in the literature. In a few cases, a 0–100-point scale was used, with various forms of presentation. However, most used some form of Likert Scale. For instance, one of the Eastern Surrey surveys, mentioned above, asked respondents to rate the relative importance of each of a list of treatments on a scale (essential/important/less important/unimportant). Aggregated results were presented either as means (without prior normalisation) or in the form of the percentage of respondents giving each type of response.

In a study which predated the one reported above, Dumfries and Galloway Health Board (1992) sought GPs' opinions to assist health service planning. A postal survey was conducted which asked respondents to rate 26 hospital and 29 community services on a five-point scale on two dimensions: quantity (1=overprovided, 5=grossly inadequate) and quality (1=excellent, 5=very poor, 6=insufficient experience). The results were presented giving the mean score of each service on each dimension and also the percentage of respondents allocating a score of 4 or 5 to a service.

As part of a project on 'Developing Consensus on the Management of Women with Breast Cancer using the Delphi Technique', conducted by Mid Downs, Worthing and

Chichester Health Authorities, the views of service users attending four DGHs and the views of a sample from the general population were obtained. Among other questions, respondents were asked to rate the importance of 15 issues raised by service providers on a 1–7 visual analogue scale. The general public were also asked to rate four aspects of service delivery (speed of access, level of specialisation, journey time, patient support), presented in the form of 16 questions giving all possible combinations of levels of the four aspects, on a 1–10 scale.

Constrained rating

Constrained rating is reported by Bowling (1993), Bowling *et al.* (1993) and Whitty (1992). However, none gives any specific name to this approach. Whitty describes an interview survey using structured questionnaires aimed at a random sample of the public in Colchester. Among other questions, respondents were asked to rate six interventions as essential, very important or not important, using each category only twice, and to rate 12 services as essential, very important, important or less important, using each category only three times. The questions were posed using show cards with a Likert-type layout. Aggregated results are presented in tabular form, showing for each option the number of respondents choosing each category. The constraint on the rating is indicated in the headings of the relevant tables. Bowling reports the use of 'constrained rating' in a major study carried out in City and Hackney where respondents, who were asked to rate 16 services as essential, very important, important or less important, were limited to using each response four times. The results were presented both in the form of the percentage of responses in each category for each service and the mean score for each service, allocating Essential =1, etc. The services were ranked according to the mean score and the resulting rankings for five different groups (public community groups, public random sample, GPs, consultants and public health doctors) were compared. The constraint on the rating is described in the methodology but not noted in the presentation of results.

Budget pie

Surprisingly, very few examples of 'standard' budget pie were found although, as discussed below, several examples of its two-option version – constant sum paired comparison – were found. As to the 'standard' budget pie approach, Honigsbaum *et al.* (1995) describe its use by the Southampton Health Commission in a priority-setting exercise where the commissioners each allocated 100 points between five criteria; their responses were combined to produce criterion weights. However, in an earlier exercise in Southampton, an attempt was made to allocate a total of £500 000 to different targets but it was found not to 'provide a clear-cut picture of priorities' (Heginbotham *et al.*, 1992). As mentioned above, Southern Derbyshire Health Authority, as part of a public consultation day, invited focus groups to allocate £100 between a set of options. However, few succeeded in this task.

Paired comparison

A few projects used some form of paired comparison, including some examples of constant sum paired comparison, a two-option version of budget pie. In the survey reported by Whitty (1992) respondents were asked to divide £1 million between: (a) ten people with severe problems and 100 people with less severe problems; (b) services for the elderly and services for children; (c) caring for old people in hospital or in their home; (d) hospital services or immunisation; (e) to have children treated in Colchester hospitals or the same treatment in London hospitals. However, apart from (e), the mean responses were fairly close to an even split. Further, between 107 (30%) and 171 (48%) respondents were unable to express a preference and gave equal amounts. It is not clear whether this resulted from resistance to the question, difficulty in responding to a question received aurally, the amount of money involved or whether it was a true reflection of respondents' values. Bowling (1993) reports the same question as (a) above being posed, but restricting the responses to giving 100%, 75%, 50%, 25% or 0% to the ten people (the remaining percentage going to the 100 people).

Seven authorities reported using the consultancy approach, Priority Search, which as part of its methodology employs scaled paired comparison. Simple paired comparisons were not much in evidence.

Simple trade-off

The simple trade-off method, which is also known as Compensation or Sacrifice, was employed in a marginal analysis study conducted by Mid Glamorgan Health Authority (Cohen, 1994), which examined the effect of altering the existing balance of expenditure between healthcare programmes. Respondents – a working group including consultants, a GP, nurses and other health staff plus representatives from the CHC and National Childbirth Trust – were first required to identify ten items for expansion and ten items for contraction. They were then asked to estimate, in terms of workload and health, the effect of 'an expansion by £100 000 for interventions on the investment list' (p.783). For the items on the disinvestment lists, the group 'was asked to imagine that a £100 000 reduction in each activity on the list of disinvestments had already occurred and what they would do if an additional £100 000 now became available'. This could involve restoring a 'disinvestment' or adding an 'investment'. This was repeated ten times. In the second stage of the project, criteria against which the interventions could be evaluated were identified (evidence of effectiveness; distance from national target; numbers of patients treated; whether the intervention was centred on people; the severity of the condition; and the extent of jurisdiction of the health authority). However, since 'the core evaluation team representing senior medical and nursing professionals, planners, general practitioners, and community health councils' (p.783) were unable to achieve a consensus on weights, all criteria were, in effect, allocated equal weights. The team then scored each proposal against these criteria and five 'clear winners' and five 'clear losers' emerged.

The marginal analysis approach, as used here, represents a specific and targeted approach to priority setting. However, although a useful and focused approach, it does require usable information about various service components and the movement of resources from one part of a service to another is frequently much more difficult in practice than it seems in theory.

Single stage versus multistage

The overwhelming majority of projects used single-stage valuation. However, a few did use some form of multistage process, including the Mid Glamorgan exercise discussed above. In an prioritisation exercise conducted by Exeter and North Devon Health Authority, which involved a range of participants including CHC members, HA members and NHS staff, participants individually ranked ten evaluation criteria 10 (highest) to 1 (lowest). These criteria included value for money, a common and worthwhile problem, evidence that the service is effective or that it works. The responses were aggregated using means of the rank 'scores' to produce criterion weights. Each service under consideration (cancer services, drug abuse, waiting lists, urinary incontinence, *in vitro* fertilisation) was then rated on a 0–100 scale against each criterion and the mean of each rating was multiplied by the criterion weight and then summed to produce a score for that service. Patient vignettes for each service were used to assist participants in their task.

In the Southampton study reported by Honigsbaum *et al.* (1995) the criterion weights resulting from the budget pie (see above) were combined with scores allocated to each of 49 options (on a 0–3 scale for each criterion) to produce a ranking of the 49 interventions. Wakefield Healthcare used the aggregated scores approach to incorporate public preferences, which had been obtained from a postal survey in which respondents had been asked to select the five top-priority services from a list of 14 types of service development. These views were then fed into an additive prioritisation 'model', with a maximum score of 50 points (public preference could score a maximum of four points; GP preference, maximum four points; degree of benefit, maximum six points; numbers involved, maximum six points; strength of research evidence, maximum nine points; prevention versus treatment, maximum nine points; appropriate setting, maximum six points; and promotion of equity, also a maximum of six points).

Postscript

From our survey and from the literature there is an overwhelming impression of ingenuity and enterprise. However, there is also evidence of studies being carried out in isolation from each other and with little knowledge of techniques developed and used elsewhere. One of the factors which prompted our original study was a concern to prevent reinvention of the wheel and to assist users to draw on the work of others.

However, the ability to learn from, and develop on, the work of others is predicated on easy access to their methodology. Regrettably, whilst some of the published articles and reports were models of clarity in presenting their methodology, many others required considerable detailed 'detective work' to ascertain their methodology and even then some methodologies remained totally opaque. Whilst in some cases this lack of clarity can be attributed to commercial confidentiality – itself a source of regret in connection with health services research – in others it appears unintended. This issue needs to be addressed if publication, whether in journals or reports, is to serve as a vehicle for the dissemination of techniques/approaches and their practical application for others to learn from.

CHAPTER EIGHT

Key concepts – the continuing debate

Tough decisions

At the outset of this text we attempted to explore the context of increased international interest in priority setting in healthcare. It is clear that many authors make the assumption that rationing is inevitable and that much stereotyped thinking follows from this basic assumption both in the use of terms and in the approaches employed.

We have tried to explore the concept of priority setting in a more detached and probing manner. Similarly, in later chapters, methods of engaging the public in priority setting have been reviewed and scrutinised in terms of their rigour and appropriateness. In this final chapter, the concept and practice of priority setting are brought together to represent our current thinking on these issues.

The first and perhaps overarching conceptual issue is that of whether rationing is inevitable. Many of the authors we have cited here preface their material with the premise that rationing is inevitable. Typically this is supported by arguments about infinite demand, governments needing to control expenditure and the cost implications of drugs, technology and an ageing population. Such comments have been repeated so often that they have acquired the status of a 'truism'. Moreover, they are frequently surrounded by macho language of 'hard choices', 'tough decisions', etc. and through such rhetoric attempt to assume the intellectual high ground of 'facing reality'. Opponents of such a position are usually described as soft, unrealistic, politically naïve or unwilling to face up to these difficult, and therefore somehow superior, decisions.

But is the position as clearcut as the rationers would have us believe?

There is little suggestion that healthcare expenditure in the UK is, or could be, at such a high level as to constitute a threat to the economy. At the same time, despite frequent talk of 'infinite demand' for healthcare, on examination there is little evidence to support that notion. Even if it were argued that there are an infinite number of procedures which, theoretically, could be carried out on marginal and hopeless cases, there is little suggestion that there would be any considerable demand for such treatment. Thus, there appears to be no absolute case that healthcare need/demand will always outstrip supply and that rationing is inevitable.

Whether or not healthcare resources, within the publicly funded sector, are insufficient to meet need/demand thus appears to be a matter of choice, not objective necessity. Perhaps the public debate should not be on 'how we should ration healthcare', as proposed by the advocates of rationing, but 'whether we wish to ration healthcare (within the NHS)'. Given that the NHS is already relatively efficient, the main focus would thus be on the overall level of resources allocated to the NHS, with a secondary focus on eliminating treatments proven to be of no benefit at all or proven to be, on balance, harmful. Despite its low standing in the OECD 'league' tables of economic performance, the UK is still, by world standards, a rich country. We need to ask not only whether we, as a society, are happy that some relatively peripheral treatments – abdominoplasty, sex change treatments and removal of wisdom teeth (Brindle, 1995b) – might be available only to those with the ability to pay but whether we, as a society, are willing to deny expensive life-saving treatment, possibly with a low probability of success, to those needing and wishing it. The public reaction to the case of Jaymee Bowen suggests that the answer might be no. Clearly, there are many cases where patients (or their advocates) refuse (further) painful 'heroic' life-saving treatment. Whilst this most frequently occurs with elderly patients, younger patients have been known to refuse further, painful, possibly near-futile treatment. However, society needs to debate whether or not it wishes to extrapolate from this and deny such treatment, even where the patient wishes to receive it.

A possible dangerous tendency to reduce the value of human life to healthcare costs can be detected in some of the comments surrounding the birth of conjoined twins, where the parents were criticised for continuing with the pregnancy because of the high costs that would be involved in treating the twins (*Observer*, 1995). If abortion on the grounds of avoiding future healthcare costs were permitted (and its legality is doubtful), would we wish to move from there and advocate, or even require, such abortions? Clearly the answer must lie in ethics and not, at least in a rich country, in economics.

Even if NHS resources are such that treatment must be 'rationed' – recalling that 'rationing' would be far less painful in the face of abundant resources than with severely restricted resources – another area of legitimate public debate is whether such rationing should be 'implicit', conducted via general priorities and global budgets, leaving clinicians and other healthcare professionals to allocate resources within those budgets, or 'explicit' with commissioners, with or without public consultation, deciding in increasingly greater detail which treatments should be provided and which should not. There is some limited evidence that the public may prefer the former (Heginbotham, 1993). Hunter (1993a, p.34) makes a very powerful case in favour of implicit rather than explicit rationing, concluding 'We should resist abandoning an admittedly imperfect though workable irrationality in favour of a spurious and possibly risky rationality'.

Finally, it is increasingly clear that the unquestioning acceptance of the necessity of rationing, with its corollary that the only question is how it should be carried out, whilst understandable for the the individual health authority or primary care group attempting to balance their budget, is leading to a climate of defeatism and is detracting both from debates about what sort of health service our society really wants and from consideration of whether rationing can be avoided or, at least, involve fewer 'hard choices'.

Nevertheless, even if the absolute need to ration healthcare is not quite as clearcut as is often implied, it is realistic to assume that competing pressures on budgets, the impossibility of delivering services simultaneously to all those needing them and competing attributes (e.g. access versus efficiency) in the way services are delivered will lead to the need to set priorities (see Box 4.1). Such priority setting might be reflected in the amount of resource attached to each service or the speed of developing in other areas, as well as in scheduling the order and speed of treatment. In addition, it is highly likely, despite the many difficulties, that the pressure to involve the public in the priority-setting process will remain or possibly intensify.

Priority setting in practice – unresolved issues

When looking at priority setting in practice, especially where there have been attempts to involve the public, the first conclusion is that there is a clear need for the dissemination of information on available techniques, as there is considerable evidence of 'reinvention of the wheel' and use of inappropriate techniques. Further, even in studies which exhibit a high degree of sophistication in sampling and statistical analysis, there is evidence that researchers are unaware of the range of techniques available for eliciting values. Indeed, several suggest that this area is in its infancy and describe their work as pioneering. Several studies claimed that their main aim was to test whether it is possible to elicit values and preferences from service users and the general public. However, although there is little need for that as there is long evidence that such value elicitation is possible, care must be taken in the interpretation of those 'values'. It should not be concluded, simply because people are willing and able to answer questions concerning values and priorities, that the 'values' thus elicited are meaningful and actually reflect the respondents' real values.

Indeed, the stability (or instability) of the public's view is illustrated by a recent study by Dolan *et al.* (1999). Using focus groups they describe a steady and consistent movement in attitudes between the first and subsequent meetings of the group. It is almost as if the uninformed public have a set of views – usually towards a rather simplistic and rigid form of priority setting – but as they acquire more information their views become closer to those of health professionals.

Many studies demonstrate considerable ingenuity in their methods of 'capturing the public' and, although the literature and study of similar public consultation exercises in other fields and in other countries will have much to teach us, problems specific to the NHS must be recognised. However, the concern expressed by some NHS staff engaged in public participation exercises about the public's level of understanding of NHS structure and the respective roles of purchasers and providers, etc. (in particular, the argument that such understanding is necessary to enable the public to participate) requires close investigation. It could be argued that it is the role of the NHS to facilitate participation and to redirect 'incorrectly' addressed messages to the appropriate level of the NHS, rather than it being the role of the public to 'communicate' with the NHS on the NHS's terms.

Few, if any, projects in the survey outlined in Chapter Seven exhibited any awareness of ethical and technical problems associated with the aggregation of individual values, although a few did use aggregation and presentation techniques designed to demonstrate the range of responses. This, however, leads on to a major question: how necessary is it to be concerned about the technical validity of methodologies used in local studies? Part of the answer must lie in the way in which the results are going to be used. On the one hand, it could be argued that if the prime objective of a study is to go through the process of involving the public – and there were repeated reports of the benefit gained from the *process* of carrying out consultation exercises with users and the wider general public – then any technical (or even ethical) lack of validity of a value elicitation exercise is of secondary importance. On the other hand, if the outcomes of such exercises are actually used to determine (or even inform) priorities and resource redeployment, it would appear essential to have regard to the validity of the methods used for eliciting and aggregating values and to ensure that those using such methods have an understanding of their implications.

This point was stressed many years ago by Hoinville and Courtenay (1979, p.175) who concluded, after ten years of conducting consultation exercises with the public, that there is no single technique or easy solution. 'Measurements have to be tailored to the application to which they will be put. Questions must be as closely linked as possible to the way the answers will be used.'

Interestingly, this point of being very clear about exactly what public involvement is to be used for is echoed by Entwistle *et al.* (1998) in their discussion of evidence-informed patient choice. Although their paper is concerned with public involvement at a different level, i.e. choices of individual patients about their own healthcare programme in the light of evidence or information provided, they point to many of the dilemmas that parallel our discussion of public involvement in determining healthcare provision for the wider population.

For example, Entwistle and her colleagues suggest that two arguments in particular justify greater public participation in decisions about their treatment. The first is that of moral obligation to provide information relevant to their choice of care. The second reason is the assumed benefits of greater rationality in decision making such as more clinically effective treatments provided, more individually appropriate healthcare offered, reduced overall expenditure and reduced litigation against healthcare professionals.

The authors point out that there is little evidence about the input of greater patient involvement but note that, just as with more population-based decisions, much of the debate quickly moves on to focus upon how such involvement should occur.

More parallels may be seen in further issues raised about how evidence-informed patient choice might be progressed. Do patients have sufficient technical knowledge? Would many patients prefer the professionals to take the decision? Would greater tension and conflict develop in the patient–doctor relationship if opposing views result from the greater information available? Are there boundaries to the content of decisions offered: an entire surgical intervention, the materials for a particular prosthesis, etc.? In this text we have also examined just such questions in terms of how public involvement in priority setting should be conducted. But perhaps the clearest and most important parallel is Entwistle *et al.*'s conclusion that any evaluation of evidence-informed patient choice must depend largely on the question of what it is aiming to achieve and, further, how the methods used interact to influence outcomes produced. We would endorse this view with respect to priority setting in general.

New Zealand is often regarded as having taken a pioneering approach to priority setting. Certainly, New Zealand's health system has been active in priority setting throughout the 1990s and other countries have sought to learn from its initiatives. However, as a case study of priority setting, and the relatively small overall population of New Zealand perhaps permits this approach, it encapsulates many of the issues, potential and uncertainties of priority setting we have identified in this text.

Edgar (1998) provides an overview of the current position of priority setting within the New Zealand health system. Given New Zealand's enthusiasm for priority setting, it is not surprising that the work of the National Health Committee is founded on the absolute assumption that rationing is inevitable (see our earlier discussion of this point in Chapter Two and in this chapter). Moreover, they then assume that decisions about health services must be as open and transparent as possible and that the general public must be involved. However, the New Zealand experience highlights a number of priority-setting dilemmas.

Priority-setting dilemmas

The first dilemma, readily acknowledged by Edgar and discussed within this text, is who are the general public and what legitimacy do they or some subsection of them have to make healthcare decisions on behalf of their fellow citizens? As Edgar (1998) suggests, 'The public is not a simple concept'. Virtually every member of the public has had some direct or indirect experience of the health service and thereby may have a variety of views about it and the services provided, not to mention the impact of media activities on these views at different points in time. The National Health Committee in New Zealand recognises that these views will be encountered in its interaction with the public and therefore it expects a range of outcomes to be reflected. However, as Spurgeon (1998) observes in commenting upon this point, the range of views is acknowledged but the processes employed seem to offer no particular way of resolving the differences.

Thus the issue of classifying what constitutes 'the public' is problematic in terms of their diversity and, more especially, in how diverse views may be reconciled. In addition the legitimacy of public decision making is exacerbated by the question of how individuals arrive at or are recruited on to relevant priority-setting panels generally. Edgar (1998, p.4) seems to reflect this unresolved concern when she says 'Striving for "a public view" on rationing may not be a sensible goal. There will always be many views, depending on the audience and the issue of the day'.

This is a commendably open and honest comment from someone heavily engaged in priority setting. It helps to move the focus to the second dilemma: what should the public participation process be about? Much of the New Zealand work, and indeed much of that in the UK, is concerned with combinations of:

- awareness raising or education
- debate about the principles
- providing and sharing information.

Only in a limited number of cases does the participation process seem to be directed to specific decision making.

This would suggest that an implicit dimension of public involvement in priority setting may be emerging whereby the 'softer' end encompasses educational and informational processes and is generally seen as positive and non-controversial. The choice of method too becomes less of an issue because it is seen as such a worthy objective that, even if the method is less than perfect, the advancement in public awareness or involvement is regarded as useful. It is at the opposite end of the priority-setting spectrum that concerns lie and technical difficulties emerge. Advocates of greater explicitness in healthcare priority setting (Ham, 1998) would seem to be operating within a hard choices, more sharply focused arena. The problem is that the approaches and methods suggested by advocates of explicit decision making are the same as those used in the 'soft' domain. However, the deficiencies of such techniques, when applied to 'hard choice' type decisions, become of increasing concern. For example, is it appropriate for decisions which disadvantage one section of the population to be taken by others when, as Edgar has pointed out, we know there will be a range of competing views? Health conditions which are extremely rare and therefore likely to be relatively under-represented and underadvocated will be very vulnerable to such a 'hard choices' approach. If we are to pursue the line of explicit priority setting, then we need to acknowledge the implicit non-democratic aspect and seek to establish some cautionary or protective measures.

Linked to the issue of the legitimacy of the content of priority-setting decisions is the third dilemma: at what level priority setting should occur. New Zealand may offer some very helpful insights here. The National Health Committee charged with the process of public involvement is in fact separated from the organisation responsible for the purchase of healthcare for particular populations. The Committee's role is to gather information and advice. This would seem to parallel emerging structures in the UK with the establishment of central bodies such as NICE (National Institute for Clinical Effectiveness) seeking to offer local health authorities and primary care groups advice on treatments and outcomes (effectiveness). This more centralist approach may offer a way out of some of the UK's more contentious but essentially localised priority-setting problems, e.g. rationing by post-code (Spurgeon, 1998).

Indeed, New Zealand has developed a value-based framework for considering whether services should be provided or not. The framework (see Box 8.1) has received wide endorsement and perhaps offers a sensible approach to where public priority setting should be focused.

Box 8.1: Framework for Rationing Decisions (National Advisory Committee, 1992)

- Benefit or effectiveness of the services
- Value for money or cost-effectiveness
- Fairness in access and use of the resource
- Consistency with communities' values

There would also appear to be a slight shift in approach in more recent priority-setting work in New Zealand which again may parallel developments in the UK such as the establishment of NICE and the growth of evidence-based medicine. The public for many reasons (lack of technical knowledge, personal involvement, different value systems) represent an emotional, highly labile and perhaps irreconcilable group and therefore more explicit priority setting faces a considerable dilemma. As guidelines, protocols of care and evidence-based medicine develop, it seems priority setting may attempt to move to a more logical/systematic/consistent basis. New Zealand has tried hard to move clinical effectiveness or clinical outcome more firmly into the priority-setting debate. Thus treatments/procedures are debated in the light of such evidence. The approach is easier to defend and appears to have attracted considerable support. It may be that there are relatively few treatments where the outcome evidence is poor and unchallenged but, at least in terms of public priority setting and effective use of public resources, it may offer a way to achieve some progress, as reducing expenditure in non-effective treatment areas may be more acceptable.

It is worth, however, recalling from the discussion in Chapter Three that even if a high degree of agreement were achieved through public involvement mechanisms outside the normal processes of representative democracy, this would not necessarily confer democratic legitimacy on those decisions. In addition, although few would oppose the elimination of treatments of no clinical effectiveness, it will be recalled from Chapter Four that moving from clinical effectiveness to cost-effectiveness – and maximising QALY gain – can pose a number of problems relating to equity, social solidarity, the 'insurance' role of the health services and, possibly most controversially, the 'rule of rescue'.

The fourth dilemma relates to the methods employed in priority setting. A recent research project (Rutt, 1997; Spurgeon, 1998) may serve to summarise this dilemma. In a priority-setting exercise over 800 respondents were asked to participate using three different methods: focus groups, survey and rapid appraisal. The important findings from this study were:

- that the methods used (all exploring the same issues) produced different priorities
- that different methods result in different levels of willingness to engage in the priority-setting task
- that a factor analysis of the data obtained using the survey approach revealed three main factors which may in themselves go some way to explaining the difficulty in resolving priority-setting issues. The factors suggested that: (i) there are varying perceptions of the appropriateness of involving the public in priority setting (Factor 1 = 22% of the variance); (ii) that views vary about the role of professionals in establishing priorities (Factor 2 = 17% of the variance); (iii) that NHS information is seen as very complex (Factor 3 = 12% of the variance).

The combination of competing views within these factors illustrates the difficulty of achieving clear priority decisions.

Who are the public?

Partly in response to this confused situation, the New Zealand National Health Committee is proposing to establish a network of skilled consumers. This parallels other approaches which aim to draw on the views of 'informed' consumers, such as citizens' juries and standing panels. Such developments may well make processes more effective and are likely to move the public view closer to the professional view. However, is that what is wanted? In many ways, as discussed in Chapter Three, is it not the public in the 'raw' that we need to involve? It may be that professionals will not agree with the views obtained or indeed that an uninformed majority may be seen as dominant or it could be that no clear consensus will be observed. But in the end that is one of the fundamental problems of priority setting.

Overview of techniques for eliciting values

Single vote

In this, the simplest of all the techniques, each respondent is given one vote to allocate to their preferred option, i.e.:

$$v_{ij} = 1 = Q_i \quad \text{for the single preferred option}$$

and

$$v_{ij} = 0 \quad \text{for all other options}$$

where:

v_{ij} is the value attributed to, or the number of 'votes' allocated to, the jth 'option' by the ith respondent

and

Q_i is the total allocation/quota available to the ith respondent.

Aggregation is normally by summing the 'votes' or 'points' allocated to each option, thus:

$$S_j = \sum_i v_{ij}$$

where S_j = group or aggregate 'score' of the jth option.

This method is widely used, including in first-past-the-post elections. However, it should be used with caution, recognising its limitations and ensuring the context is appropriate. It simply permits respondents to identify their single preferred option:

respondents are not permitted to express intensity of preference (being forced to allocate 100% of their 'vote' to their first choice and 0% to all other options) and thus no information is elicited on the relationship between the preferred option and the remaining options, nor the relationships between the remaining options. However, although there is inter-respondent equity in that all respondents have the same number of 'votes' (one), simple aggregation can prove misleading where there are more than two options. The introduction of an additional option can change the 'winning' option, even though no individual changes their preference among the original options, i.e. it violates Arrow's Condition 3 (independence of irrelevant alternatives).

Multiple vote

With the multiple vote, each respondent is given k votes to allocate singly to each of their k preferred options, thus:

$$v_{ij} = 1 = \frac{Q_i}{k} \quad \text{for each of the } k \text{ preferred options}$$

and

$$v_{ij} = 0 \quad \text{for all other options } (\textit{all other notation as above}).$$

As with the single vote, aggregation is normally by summing the 'votes' or 'points' allocated to each option, thus:

$$S_j = \sum_i v_{ij}$$

Although this is again a simple technique, it must be treated with caution. Respondents are unable to indicate intensity of preference, as they are required to allocate equal 'points' or 'scores' to each of their k preferred options, with zero allocation to their $(k+1)^{th}$ and subsequent preferences. There is inter-respondent equity, as all respondents are allocated an equal number (k) of 'votes'. However, there is potential for strategic voting. Further, if respondents are forced to use all k 'votes', 'slate' voting by a group can dominate the result.

Ranking

With this ubiquitous and deceptively simple technique, each respondent is asked to rank all or the top r options in order of preference. Left at that – an ordinal expression of an individual's preferences – the technique is relatively unproblematic. However, problems arise when attempting to aggregate the preferences of different individuals.

There are a number of different approaches to such aggregation – Jensen (1986) discusses and compares at least five different methods and variants.

The approach found most frequently in health service studies involves converting the ordinal rank positions to 'scores'.[*] Thus:

$v_{ij} = 1$ for the ith respondent's first choice
$v_{ij} = 2$ for the ith respondent's second choice, etc.

and

$Q_i = \dfrac{r\,(r+1)}{2}$ 'points', where $r =$ number of options to be ranked.

Thus respondents are 'assumed' to have given equal intervals between each of the options and are 'deemed' to have given:

$\dfrac{1}{Q_i}$ or $\dfrac{1}{r(r+1)/2}$ share of their 'vote' to their first choice,

$\dfrac{2}{Q_i}$ or $\dfrac{2}{r(r+1)/2}$ to their second choice, and so on.

Therefore, although respondents are not invited to express their intensity of preference for the options, this 'scoring' methodology implicitly imposes an intensity of preference score on their choices. Aggregation is performed by summing the resulting 'scores' for each option as above, thus:

$$S_j = \sum_i v_{ij}$$

Frequently, S_j is divided by the number of respondents to determine the 'mean rank position' of the jth option. The results are often presented in the form of aggregate or group rankings of the options.

Sometimes the rank positions are reversed before converting to 'scores', i.e. each individual respondent's first preference is allocated r 'points', the second $(r-1)$ 'points', etc., with the lowest ranked option allocated 1 'point'. Aggregated scores are calculated from sums or means as above. A variant of this is the Borda count (Bonner, 1986, p.81; McLean, 1987, p.162), where the first-placed option is allocated $(r-1)$ 'points', the second-placed $(r-2)$ and so on, with the lowest ranked option receiving 0 'points'. Aggregated scores – the *Borda count* or *Borda scores* – are obtained, as above, by summing the scores for each option across all respondents.

However, despite the fact that these scoring methods are claimed to have some advantages over the two voting methods discussed above, in that they use information (the rank positions) about all the options, they pose a number of problems. First, they

---

[*] The Borda-Kendall method (Jensen, 1986).

require that each respondent ranks all the options. Second, in addition to, or rather because of, the implied assumption of equal intervals between options with the resulting imposed 'intensity of preference', they can be vulnerable to violating Arrow's Condition 3 (independence of irrelevant alternatives) in that the inclusion of an additional option, which does not alter any individual's ranking of the original options, can alter the aggregate or group rank positions of the original options (Box 2: Goodman and Markowitz, 1952). This applies regardless of whether rank positions are simply translated into 'scores' or whether one of the reverse-score methods is used.

Clearly, many of the problems with ranking occur as a result of 'translating' ordinal data into cardinal data. Among other things, the resulting 'scores', especially with the 'reverse' methods, are affected by the number of options ranked. This is a particular problem if the resulting scores are treated as if they have ratio properties.

Sometimes the results of a ranking exercise are presented in the form of the number of times (or the percentage of times) each option is ranked first. The method then, in effect, becomes the single vote technique.

Despite the many problems associated with it, ranking is widely used to determine people's preferences. As noted above, left at that – as an ordinal ranking of individuals' preferences – it poses few problems. However, the implications of converting rank positions to 'scores' (by whatever method) and then performing arithmetic manipulation of these scores should be fully understood and taken into account. In many instances, it will be realised that the disadvantages outweigh the initial simplicity of the technique and that more suitable techniques, for instance budget pie or a rating method, should be adopted.

Budget pie (Clark, 1974, 1976)

This method, also known as *constant sum measurement* (Hauser and Shugan, 1980), the *point voting system* (Brown and Jackson, 1978), a *coupon scale* (Strauss and Hughes, 1976) and the *method of marks* (Dodgson, 1873, reprinted 1958), is extremely simple but rather underused. Respondents are allocated a fixed total or quota of votes, points or money which they may allocate in any combinations and quantities to a set of competing options, values, objectives or proposals, i.e.:

v_{ij} (*as defined above*) can take any value, subject to

$$\sum_j v_{ij} = Q_i$$

As in the two voting systems above, aggregation is by summation, i.e.:

$$S_j = \sum_i v_{ij}$$

Thus, within the constraints of their total allocation or allowance, respondents are able to express their intensity of preference for the different options and the 'values' obtained are cardinal rather than ordinal. Respondents are normally allowed equal numbers of votes (Q) but, where appropriate, unequal allowances can be made. Although aggregation of values can never be entirely unproblematic, the budget pie does avoid many of the problems associated with aggregation. The approach lends itself to many different methods of presentation. Respondents can be given their allowance in the form of points, votes, poker chips, pie slices and money. The number of units allowed to each respondent should be sufficient to permit reasonably fine adjustment to their valuations, but not so excessive as to overwhelm them. A particular issue arises when using money. Small sums may be unrealistic whilst, in some contexts, realistic amounts may be outside the normal experience of respondents.

As mentioned above, this method is simple to use, both in self-completion questionnaires and in interviews. However, it is vastly underused compared with some other techniques which pose far more technical problems. It is appropriate when options are in competition, but not when they are mutually exclusive.

Scoring/rating

Each respondent is asked to give a score/mark/rating (usually within a defined range) to each option independently. Thus, v_{ij} (as defined above) can take any value within the given range.

Respondents are thus permitted to indicate their intensity of preference or value for each option, although the degree of definition allowed will depend on the range of scores permitted. As presented, the method is unconstrained: respondents do not have to trade-off between options. However, the values given by each respondent are sometimes normalised, which has the effect of implicitly forcing a trade-off.

As above, aggregation is usually by summation across all respondents for each option, thus:

$$S_j = \sum_i v_{ij}$$

If the initial scores are used (i.e. without normalisation) this results in unequal weighting between respondents since $\sum_j v_{ij}$ may be different for each respondent.

However, if the scores have been normalised, the weighting for respondents will be equal. Whether or not the scores allocated by each individual should be normalised, either to force a trade-off implicitly and/or to secure equal weighting between respondents, will depend on the nature of the options (e.g. are they in competition?) and the nature of the problem (e.g. is it reasonable for a respondent who rates options higher than another effectively to have a greater weighting in the aggregated result?).

This technique is transparent to users and, although respondents can find the task difficult, it does lend itself to use with self-completion questionnaires as well as interviews and group situations with facilitators.

Scaling

Likert Scale

This technique is similar to the above in that, for each option, respondents are asked to select a position on a 'scale' with five or more 'points'. The 'points' on the scale are usually expressed as categories (e.g. strongly agree to strongly disagree). The scale 'points' or positions are frequently converted into scores (usually equidistant). Thus, respondents are permitted to express intensity of preference but only within the limitations of the 'scale', which may or may not be revealed to respondents in numerical form.

As noted above, it is possible to extend the scale to 7, 9, 11 or even more. However, when going beyond five points it is probably wise not to try to provide precise linguistic versions of the numerical scale since this introduces the variability of interpretation of language and thereby potential bias.

Debate exists about the middle position in such unequal scales. Some advocate eliminating the middle position as it can be used as an 'opt-out'. However, the opposite view is that the neutral position is for some people a valid position and forcing them into a pro or anti stance is inappropriate. Ultimately it is always possible to dichotomise the data, retrospectively omit the middle position and combine the for and against scores.

If aggregation is carried out by summing the scores for each option as above:

$$S_j = \sum_i v_{ij}$$

there will be inter-respondent inequity in that $\sum_j v_{ij}$ may be different for each respondent.

However, although in the context of priority setting the Likert Scale can readily produce an average score for particular treatment options, the degree of spread around the average is an important calculation for this represents individuals who hold quite different views in potentially opposing directions.

As an alternative, aggregation is frequently carried out by presenting the full range of responses for each option (i.e. the number or percentage 'strongly agreeing', etc.), which is relatively unproblematic.

This technique is relatively easy to use, but requires careful research design.

Although it is fairly transparent to both users and respondents, the imposition of numerical 'scores' on categories can prove misleading.

Visual analogue scale (VAS)

This is a variant of the scoring/rating method above. Instead of being asked to give a 'score' for each option, respondents are asked to indicate the value they attribute to each option on a visual scale (usually marked 0–10 or 0–100). The scale is sometimes presented in a 'thermometer' format. Some variants of this latter method require that the lowest valued option is scored 0 and the highest valued option is scored 100.

This presentation is considered easier for respondents than simple 'scoring' and there is some evidence that it produces a greater spread of values. Otherwise, all the points made above in respect of scoring or rating apply here.

Delphi

'Delphi may be characterised as a method for structuring a group communication process so that the process is effective in allowing a group of individuals, as a whole, to deal with a complex problem' (Linstone and Turoff, 1975, p.3). The Delphi technique originated with technological (long-term) forecasting in the 1960s. The basic elements of the original approach were that respondents (often identified experts in the field) were asked (usually individually) to estimate the date by which an event (e.g. landing a man on the moon) would occur or to estimate the probability of that event occurring by a specific date. The responses were collated into a histogram/bar chart and fed back to the respondents. Although each individual was informed where their own response lay on the histogram, all other responses were anonymous. In a 'classic' Delphi study, successive rounds would be held with respondents being asked if they wished to revise their estimate in the light of the aggregated responses. At some point, often after two or three rounds, those who were still outliers might be invited by the researchers to explain the reasoning behind their responses.

Claimed advantages of this approach are that it taps into collective expertise, but that the method of collecting and collating the data avoids the disadvantages of group processes where the most senior or the most vocal might dominate. The effect of successive rounds may be to produce consensus, although some question whether the result is true consensus. It should be noted that not all Delphi studies aim to achieve consensus. An Expert Delphi may be more concerned with eliciting the 'correct' result from an outlier than to achieve an 'incorrect' consensus.

The approach has been adapted for use with public consultation in a variety of ways. As well as, or instead of, estimating the probability of an event occurring, respondents may be asked to estimate the importance of an option, to place a value on it or to estimate its impact. The responses obtained are normally presented in the histogram format. Depending on the nature of the study, successive rounds may or may not be used and persistent outliers may or may not be invited to explain their reasoning.

Although not widely used in public consultation, this approach has proved very adaptable and flexible. Since one of its basic characteristics is individual, anonymous responses, it is particularly suited to use with self-completion questionnaires. However, the use of successive rounds might prove difficult with a large-scale population-based study. The method of presentation avoids most of the problems normally associated with aggregation. However, as suggested above, attempts to achieve consensus through successive rounds have proved controversial.

Simple paired comparison

With this method, also known as *dominance preference* and *discrete choice*, respondents are asked to state their preference between each pair of options. Respondents are thus presented with a constrained choice, but are unable to indicate their intensity of preference. In general, the method is easy for respondents to use, but a very large number of comparisons are required if there are more than a few options involved. It can be used with both self-completion questionnaires and interviews.

If the expressed preferences are converted into a ranking of the options for each individual, the effects of aggregation are the same as for ranking, as discussed above. If aggregation is carried out on the responses for each pair of options, e.g. by group voting on each pair, the voting paradox may prove a problem.

Paired comparison is frequently used as part of, or in conjunction with, another methodology.

Weighted paired comparison

With this method, also known as ratio scale preference, respondents indicate their degree of preference between each pair of options. Thus:

$$a_{jk} = \frac{v_{ij}}{v_{ik}}$$

where a_{jk} is the weight given to the jth option relative to the kth by the ith respondent.

Consistency is usually assumed in that:

$$a_{kj} = \frac{1}{a_{jk}}$$

The responses need complex transformation (such as that used with AHP, see below) to obtain option or attribute values. The method is implicit and unconstrained and allows respondents to indicate intensity of preference. As with simple paired comparison, a very large number of comparisons are required if there are more than a few options. Although the method is usually relatively easy for respondents to use, the subsequent transformation of responses to obtain option values or scores can mean that the approach is not very transparent. Inter-respondent inequity can occur if the resulting values for each option are summed, unless the values for each respondent are first normalised.

Constant sum paired comparison

Respondents are given a budget of money or points to allocate between two options. This is a two-option variant of budget pie, which is claimed to be easier to use (Hauser and Shugan, 1980). As with the budget pie (discussed above), it offers a constrained (trade-off) choice and permits respondents to indicate intensity of preference. Aggregation, which is normally by summing the allocation given to each option, is relatively unproblematic and results in inter-respondent equity. The method is generally transparent and easy to use, but there can be a large number of comparisons if more than a few options are offered.

Variants of this method limit the set of permitted responses, thus limiting respondents' expression of intensity of preference. Such variants may, in effect, be similar to simple paired comparison or, in some cases, weighted paired comparison.

Scaled paired comparison

Respondents indicate, on a scale, their relative preference between two options. Although this method has some similarities to weighted paired comparison, it is generally less transparent. Option values are computed from the responses by complex method (e.g. priority search or conjoint analysis, see below). With some methods of conversion to option values, this method is a special case of constant sum paired comparison.

This method offers respondents a constrained choice and permits them to indicate intensity of preference. Although it is easy for respondents to use, the complex transformation means that the method is not very transparent and is sometimes not fully understood by users.

Depending on the method of analysis (transformation), there is normally equity between respondents.

Analytical hierarchy process (AHP) (Saaty, 1977)

This method has two distinctive features: the presentation of the hierarchy of decision making (it is a multistage method) and the method of eliciting values or determining weights.

The methodology for eliciting values and determining weights is a form of weighted paired comparison, as described above. Where *n* elements are to be compared, a matrix:

$$A = (a_{jk}), (j,k = 1,2,....n)$$

of relative weights is created (usually for each respondent) by posing weighted pairwise comparison questions of the form 'Which of elements j and k is the more important and by how much?'. The relative importance is presented in a verbal scale from 'equal importance' to 'absolute importance', which is converted to a numerical scale 1, 3, 7, 9. The pairwise questions can be adapted to suit the context; for instance, 'Which is more important?' can be changed to 'Which is most likely to succeed?'. No consistency in responses is assumed, other than setting $a_{kj}= 1/a_{jk}$. The normalised principal eigenvector of the paired comparison matrix gives the relative weights of the elements being compared. Consistency is tested using a consistency index and consistency ratio (Saaty and Alexander, 1980).

The basic structure of the hierarchy is similar to other decision systems in that it consists of an overall objective broken down into a number of attributes or criteria. These attributes or criteria (elements) are valued relative to each other to determine weights (using the matrix described above). The options (elements) under consideration are then valued relative to each other for these criteria/attributes in turn (again using the pairwise matrix described above). Assuming a two-stage model, the 'score' for each option is the product of the criterion weight and the option's (relative) performance on that criterion. Where appropriate, further levels of the hierarchy can be used.

Respondents usually find the weighted pairwise questions easy to answer (but as with all paired comparison methods, where there are more than a very few options, there can be a large number of comparisons) and the representation of the hierarchy is usually easily understood. Although the calculation of the option scores is not transparent, there are two simple (transparent) methods for finding an approximation to the vector of weights, which enable the underlying working of the methodology to be easily explained to users and, if relevant, to respondents. AHP is now normally used with specialist software,* which aids data input, calculates the weights using the principal eigenvector, permits sensitivity analysis and allows a variety of graphical presentations. Respondents frequently interact with the software and thus the method is normally used with individuals and groups of respondents in person. However, Choi

---

*Two of the leading software packages for AHP are Expert Choice™ and HIPRE-3+.

et al. (1994) report a study using self-completion questionnaires to elicit responses to the pairwise comparisons.

Conjoint analysis (Ryan, 1996b)

In this method, respondents are presented with multi-attribute options, each option having a different 'mix' of values of the relevant attributes. Respondents are asked to rank or rate the options or to choose between pairs of options using weighted or scaled paired comparisons or simple discrete choice. The latter is claimed to be consistent with random utility theory (Ryan and Hughes, 1997) and thus of especial interest to economists. The resulting choices are then analysed using multiple regression to determine coefficients or weights for each attribute.

With the simple paired comparison (discrete choice), respondents are unable to indicate intensity of preference. With the other choice methods, respondents can indicate intensity of preference in different degrees. Inter-respondent aggregation is implicit in the multiple regression analysis used to obtain the coefficients for attributes.

Although respondents usually find the method easy to use, the methodology is implicit and not very transparent, even sometimes to users. Because of the very large number of options possible for every combination of attribute values, the number of options used is usually reduced to a small, normally non-dominated, set to make the number of comparisons viable and, it is claimed, to ensure the absence of multi-collinearity.

Measure of value (based on Churchman and Ackoff, 1954)

With this two-stage method, respondents first rank attributes and then are offered a series of simple paired comparisons between a single higher valued attribute and a combination of lower valued attributes, e.g. the respondent is offered the choice between:

$$c_{i1} \text{ and } c_{i2} + c_{i3} + c_{i4} + c_{i5}$$

where c_{i1} is the attribute (criterion) ranked first by the ith respondent
and c_{i2} is the attribute (criterion) ranked second, and so on.

If the combination of lower valued attributes is preferred, the lowest valued is omitted and the new comparison offered thus:

$$c_{i1} \text{ versus } c_{i2} + c_{i3} + c_{i4}$$

This process is continued until either the single higher ranked attribute (LHS) is chosen or only two attributes remain in the RHS 'combination'. The process is then repeated comparing c_{i2} with combinations of lower ranked attributes and so on.

Values of the attributes are assigned in accordance with the responses to the paired comparisons. The values thus assigned are presented to the respondent who is invited to make adjustments until they are satisfied the assigned values reflect their values. The options under consideration are then rated according to their performance against each attribute/criterion. The attribute values are then used as weights in an additive model to produce 'effectiveness' scores for each option.

In a one-stage variant of this approach, the first (successive paired comparison) stage of this method has been used to value options directly, rather than valuing attributes to act as weights in a two-stage model.

The way the combinations of attributes are presented effectively permits respondents to indicate intensity of preference. Unless the attribute values are normalised, the choices are effectively unconstrained, despite the fact that constrained choices are offered. Aggregation can prove problematic. Group 'voting' on each decision choice can lead to problems with the voting paradox. If values are obtained for each individual and then summed, inter-respondent inequity can result unless the values are normalised. Respondents find the method easy to use but not very transparent. The method needs respondents/researcher (or computer) interaction and would thus be inappropriate for use with self-completion questionnaires. There is little evidence of recent use of this method.

Time trade-off (Dolan *et al.*, 1995)

Respondents are asked to choose between a higher state of health for a shorter period or a lower state of health for a longer period. The periods in each state of health may be adjusted until the respondent is indifferent. In an alternative formulation the respondent is asked how much time they are prepared to lose (trade-off) from their life in order to move from a lower state of health to perfect health. Values for each health state are computed from the responses.

This method is explicit and fairly transparent. It offers constrained choices and allows respondents to indicate intensity of preference. Aggregation is usually carried out by computing mean responses, which may lead to difficulties of interpretation. There is, however, evidence of respondent reluctance to trade even small amounts of time (life) in order to attain perfect health.

Standard gamble (Drummond *et al.*, 1987, pp.126–8)

Respondents are offered a gamble between certainty of state of health S and $(1-p)$ probability of perfect health with p probability of death. The value of p is adjusted until the respondent is indifferent between the choices. The value of health state S relative to perfect health and death is determined from the value of p.

This method is implicit and constrained. It is not very transparent but it allows respondents to indicate intensity of preference. Aggregation is usually by computing mean values. Although one of the claimed advantages of this method is that it incorporates the notion of risk, there is considerable research evidence that respondents have difficulty dealing with probabilities, especially very low probabilities. There is also some evidence of a reluctance to accept even a small risk of death. This method is widely used by economists in many contexts.

Willingness to pay (WTP) (Donaldson *et al.*, 1997; O'Brien and
Viramontes, 1994)

Respondents are asked to indicate how much they would be willing to pay for a product or a service or how much more they would pay for some change in service. The question can be posed as open-ended, i.e. respondents are asked to write in an amount, or closed, where respondents are asked if they would be prepared to pay specific sums of money.

This approach allows respondents to indicate relative intensity of preference but inter-respondent comparison is difficult because responses may be affected by disposable income. Although the method incorporates the notion of sacrifice, respondents are effectively faced with an unconstrained choice.

Aggregation is usually by addition or calculation of means. Inter-respondent equity is compromised by differential 'purchasing power' and the fact that decisions are effectively unconstrained. In order to overcome the former problem, some attempts have been made to weight responses according to income (Donaldson, 1995).

The method is fairly transparent but it cannot deal with joint products. When applied to public health services, problems of differential purchasing power would appear insuperable. There is also some evidence of resistance from respondents when asked about WTP in connection with 'free' health services.

Qualitative discriminant process (Bryson *et al.*, 1994)

This approach, which uses vague real numbers (VRN), is claimed to address some of the problems associated with existing group support systems, especially their 'inability to deal with vagueness of human decision makers in articulating preferences ... [and] ... problems in aggregating individual preferences into meaningful group preference'.

Respondents assign options to broad categories on each criterion, then to subcategories within each category and then to sub-subcategories within those. If two or more options exist in any sub-subcategory, respondents are asked to rank them. Thus respondents appear to be given some ability to indicate intensity of preference and are constrained to some extent.

In attempting to determine group preferences, the facilitator determines if there is a sufficient degree of consensus. If not, the facilitator informs the decision makers and they repeat the individual procedures 'if they feel another round would improve the outcome'. The facilitator then generates an LP (linear programme), with the objective function to minimise difference between the 'group' score for each option and that given by each individual.

The approach does not appear to be very transparent, especially to respondents. It does produce group results (i.e. point estimates for each option), but facilitators should 'present each decision maker with his/her vector of scores'. As with most other techniques, the aggregation method will probably work better where there is a reasonable degree of consensus, but not where the preferences of the individuals are very different. The basic method for eliciting individual preferences may also prove useful in itself, i.e. without aggregation to produce group preferences.

Simple trade-off

In this compensation or 'sacrifice' method, respondents are presented with the *status quo* (for instance, the current allocation of resources to services) and are asked to indicate which services they consider should have increased expenditure and, at the same time, to indicate an equivalent number of services for reduced expenditure.

This method is explicit and faces respondents with a constrained (trade-off) choice, but respondents cannot fully indicate intensity of preference. Aggregation is usually by summing, for each service, the number of respondents indicating increased expenditure and, separately, the number of respondents indicating reduced expenditure. The method is transparent and easy for respondents to use. However, it does not easily produce cardinal valuations of options or service changes. Hoinville and Courtenay (1979) describe a more sophisticated version, the priority evaluator, which is similar to budget pie.

Priority search

In the initial stage of this procedure a series of focus groups are held, from which a list of 14–42 services and attributes (mixed in the same list) is drawn up. Respondents are then asked to indicate on a scale (scaled paired comparison, see above) their preference between a limited number of pairs (each attribute/service appears three times in the comparisons). Rankings of the services and attributes for each individual respondent are produced via commercial computer program. (The methodology is claimed to be based on personal construct theory (Kelly, 1963) but the actual algorithm used appears to be commercially confidential.)

The method is implicit and constrained, but allows respondents to indicate their intensity of preference in respect of the limited number of choices offered. The methodology is not very transparent. Respondents find making the comparisons fairly easy, but there are a large number of comparison choices to make, despite the fact that each item appears only three times.

Two main methods of aggregation to produce group values are used, both apparently resulting in inter-respondent equity. One method of aggregation is simply by calculating the means of the rank positions (see ranking, discussed above). Another method produces 'scores' for each item (service or attribute) derived from the percentage of times that item appears in the top one-third rank positions minus the percentage of times it appears in the bottom one-third rank positions. Responses are also sometimes presented in a Delphi-type format.

Constrained rating

This method appears to have been developed to overcome problems when respondents found it difficult to make a complete ranking of 12–16 options (Bowling, 1993, p.16). Respondents are asked to allocate a 'budget' of, say, four 'very importants' (VI), four 'quite importants' (QI) and four 'not importants' (NI) between 12 options. Scores are allocated, for example, VI=3 points, QI=2 points, NI=1 point. Thus, respondents must allocate:

$$\frac{1}{p(q+1)/2}$$ share of their 'vote' (allowance) to each of their first set of p choices

$$\frac{q-1}{pq(q+1)/2}$$ share to each of their second set of p choices

$$\frac{q-2}{pq(q+1)/2}$$ share to each of their third set of p choices, and so on

where p = number of choices allowed in each category
      q = number of categories of choices

and $Q_i = pq(q+1)/2$ (*notation as above*).

In an alternative formulation, respondents were presented with a format resembling a four-point Likert Scale (essential; very important; important; less important). Respondents were asked to rate each of 16 items on this scale, but with a 'budget' of four 'essentials', four 'very importants', four 'importants' and four 'less importants'. Points were allocated – 'essential' = 1 point to 'less important' = 4 points – and aggregation was carried out by calculating mean scores and ranking items on the basis of these scores (Bowling, 1993).

This method appears to be relatively easy for respondents to use but, although in one format it visually resembles a Likert Scale, it is effectively a constrained budget pie. Respondents have some limited scope to indicate intensity of preference but the scoring system forces fixed intensity allocations. The aggregation method yields inter-respondent equity, but the hybrid nature of the approach may throw up a number of aggregation problems. Although superficially transparent to respondents, the approach may not be very transparent as respondents may be misled by the presentation methods and because the conversion 'scale' is not usually presented. Users may not understand the implications of the technique.

Aggregated scores

This is essentially a two-stage (multi-criterion) model presented to respondents as a single-stage model. Respondents are asked to score the 'performance' of each option on a unique scale for each attribute (e.g. 0–3, 1–5). Thus, the range of possible values of v_{ij} is different for each j. The value or score of each option is calculated by summing the scores given for each attribute.

Respondents are permitted to indicate 'intensity' of 'performance', but they are not normally permitted to influence the attribute weights (i.e. the maximum permitted scores for each attribute). Choices are effectively unconstrained but that may be appropriate as it is normally performance that is being scored. Values are usually summed over all respondents to produce aggregated responses, which may result in inter-respondent inequity. The method is easy to use, but is not very transparent as respondents (and users) may be misled by the pre-assigned attribute values/weights. The implications of this additive model do not always appear to be understood by users.

References

Aaron H (1992) The Oregon Experiment. In: MA Strosberg *et al.* (eds) *Rationing America's Medical Care: The Oregon Plan and Beyond*. The Brookings Institution, Washington DC. pp. 107–14.

Aaron H and Schwartz WB (1990) Rationing health-care – the choice before us. *Science*. **247**(4941): 418–22.

Abelson J, Lomas J, Eyles J, Birch S and Veenstra G (1995) Does the community want devolved authority? Results from deliberative polling in Ontario. *Canadian Medical Association Journal*. **153**: 403–12.

ACHCEW (1993) *Rationing Health Care – Should Community Health Councils Help?* Health News Briefing. Association of Community Health Councils for England and Wales, London.

Algie J, Mallen G and Foster W (1983) Financial cutback decisions by priority scaling. *Journal of Management Studies*. **20**(2): 233–60.

Appelbaum PS (1993) Must we forgo informed consent to control health care costs? A response to Mark A Hall. *Milbank Quarterly*. **71**(4): 669–76.

Appleby J (1995) *Acting on the Evidence: a review of clinical effectiveness: sources of information, dissemination and implementation*. National Association of Health Authorities and Trusts, Birmingham.

Arcangelo V (1994) Should age be a criterion for rationing health care? *Nursing Forum* (New Jersey). **29**(1): 25–9.

Arnstein S (1969) A ladder of citizen participation in the USA. *Journal of the American Institute of Planners*. **35**: 216–24.

Arnstein S (1971) Eight rungs on the ladders of citizen participation. In: ES Cahn and BA Passett (eds) *Citizen Participation*, Praeger, London.

Arrow KJ (1963) *Social Choice and Individual Values*, 2nd edn. Wiley, Chichester.

Ast DB (1978) Prevention and the power of consumers (editorial). *American Journal of Public Health*. **68**: 15–16.

Audit Commission (1996) *What the Doctor Ordered*. HMSO, London.

Baker R (1993) Visibility and the just allocation of health care: a study of age-rationing in the British National Health Service. *Health Care Analysis*. **1**(2): 139–50.

Bard JF (1992) A comparison of the analytic hierarchy process with multiattribute utility-theory – a case-study. *IIE Transactions*. **24**(5): 111–21.

Baumol WJ (1993) Health care, education and the cost of disease: a looming crisis for public choice. *Public Choice.* **77**(1): 17.

Baumol WJ (1995) Health care as a handicraft industry. OHE Annual Lecture. OHE, London.

Bombardier C, Wolfson AD, Sinclair AJ and McGeer A (1982) Comparison of three preference measurement methodologies in the evaluation of a functional status index. In: R Deber and G Thompson (eds) *Choices in Health Care: Decision Making and Evaluation of Effectiveness.* University of Toronto Press, Toronto.

Bone MR, Bebbington AC, Jagger C, Morgan K and Nicolaas G (1995) *Health Expectancy and Its Uses.* HMSO, London.

Bonner J (1986) *Politics, Economics and Welfare.* Wheatsheaf Books, Brighton.

Boseley S (1995) Never give up, says leukaemia girl. *The Guardian,* 26 October.

Bowie C, Richardson A and Sykes W (1995) Consulting the public about health service priorities. *British Medical Journal.* **311**(7013): 1155–8.

Bowling A (1993) *What People Say about Prioritising Health Services.* King's Fund Centre, London.

Bowling A, Jacobson B and Southgate L (1993) Explorations in consultation of the public and health professionals on priority setting in an Inner London Health District. *Social Science and Medicine.* **37**(7): 851–7.

Brannigan M (1993) Oregon's experiment. *Health Care Analysis.* **1**(1): 15–32.

Brindle D (1995a) Fresh limits on NHS feared – surgery rationing plan may spread. *The Guardian,* 30 August.

Brindle D (1995b) NHS treatments ruled out by cost. *The Guardian,* 27 September.

Brindle D (1995c) Secret summit plans rationing for NHS. *The Guardian,* 27 October.

Brooks DG and O'Leary TJ (1983) A comparison of encoding techniques. *OMEGA.* **11**(1): 49–55.

Brown CV and Jackson PM (1978) *Public Sector Economics.* Martin Robertson, Oxford, Chapter 4.

Brown LD (1991) The national politics of Oregon's rationing plan. *Health Affairs.* **10**(2): 28–51.

Bryson N, Ngwenyama OK and Mobolurin A (1994) A qualitative discriminant process for scoring and ranking in group support systems. *Information Processing and Management.* **30**(3): 389–405.

Buede DM and Maxwell DT (1995) Rank disagreement: a comparison of multi-criteria methodologies. *Journal of Multi-criteria Decision Analysis.* **4**(1): 1–21.

Bull AR (1991) Problems of prioritisation and our duty to care. *Journal of Management in Medicine.* **5**(4): 35–9.

Califano JA (1992) Rationing health-care – the unnecessary solution. *University of Pennsylvania Law Review.* **140**(5): 1525–38.

Callahan D (1987) *Setting Limits: Medical Goals in an Aging Society.* Simon and Schuster, New York.

Callahan D (1991) Ethics and priority setting in Oregon. *Health Affairs.* **10**(2): 78–87.

Callahan D (1993) Should health care for the elderly be rationed?. *Coronary Artery Disease.* **4**(4): 393–4.

Calnan M (1995) Citizens views on health care. *Journal of Management in Medicine.* **9**(4): 17–23.

Camasso MJ and Dick J (1993) Using multiattribute utility theory as a priority-setting tool in human services planning. *Evaluation and Program Planning.* **16**(4): 295–304.

Campanelli P (1995) Minimising non-response before it happens: what can be done. *Survey Methods Bulletin.* **37**: 35–7.

Carr-Hill RA (1989) Assumptions of the QALY procedure. *Social Science and Medicine.* **29**(3): 469–77.

Choi HA, Suh EH and Suh CK (1994) Analytic hierarchy process: it can work for group decision support systems. *Computers and Industrial Engineering.* **27**(1/4): 167–71.

Christensen DB and Wertheimer AI (1976) Consumer action in health care. *Public Health Report.* **91**: 406–11.

Churchman CW and Ackoff RL (1954) An approximate measure of value. *Operations Research.* **2**(2): 172–81.

Clark TN (1974) Can you cut a budget pie? *Policy and Politics.* **3**(2): 3–31.

Clark TN (1976) Modes of collective decision-making: eight criteria for evaluation of representatives, referenda, participation and surveys. *Policy and Politics,* 4: 13–22.

Clayton M (1998) Rationing in health care. *Journal of Health Services Research Policy.* **3**(1): 58–9.

Cohen D (1994) Marginal analysis in practice: an alternative to needs assessment for contracting for health care. *British Medical Journal.* **309**: 781–4.

Cooper MH (1995) Core services and the New Zealand health reforms. *British Medical Bulletin.* **51**(4): 799–807.

Cooper TL (1979) The hidden price tag: participation costs and health planning. *American Journal of Public Health.* **69**(4): 368–74.

Coote A (1993) Public participation in decisions about health care. *Critical Public Health.* **4**(1): 36–49.

Coote A and Hunter D (1996) *New Agenda for Health.* Institute for Public Policy Research, London

Coote A and Lenaghan J (1997) *Citizens' Juries: Theory into Practice.* Institute for Public Policy Research, London.

Courtenay G and Field J (1975) *South Yorkshire Structure Plan – Public Attitude Survey.* Social and Community Planning Research, London.

Crawshaw R (1990) Health-care rationing. *Science.* **248**(4956): 662–3.

Culyer AJ and Wagstaff A (1993) Equity and equality in health and health care. *Journal of Health Economics.* **12**(4): 431–57.

Cumming J (1994) Core services and priority setting: the New Zealand experience. *Health Policy.* **29**: 41–60.

Daniels N (1985) *Just Health Care.* Cambridge University Press, Cambridge.

Daniels N (1991) Is the Oregon rationing plan fair? *Journal of the American Medical Association.* **265**(17): 2232–5.

Deber RB and Geol V (1990) Using explicit decision rules to manage issues of justice, risk and ethics in decision analysis: when is it not rational to maximise expected utility? *Medical Decision Making.* **10**(3): 181–94.

Defever M (1991) Long term care: the case of the elderly. *Health Policy.* **19**(1): 1–18.

Dicker A and Armstrong D (1995) Patients' views of priority setting in health care: an interview survey in one practice. *British Medical Journal.* **311**(7013): 1137–9.

Dickinson AL (1979) Getting the best value from additional resources. *Hospital and Health Services Review.* **April**: 127–9.

Dobson J (1993) Labour suggests housing list style approach to hospital waiting time. *Health Service Journal.* **103**(5342): 7.

Dodd FJ and Donegan HA (1995) Comparison of prioritization techniques using inter-hierarchy mappings. *Journal of the Operational Research Society.* **46**(4): 492–8.

Dodgson CL (Lewis Carroll) (1873) A discussion of the Various methods of Procedures in Conducting Elections, privately printed, Oxford. Reprinted in Black D (1958) *The Theory of Committees and Elections.* Cambridge University Press, Cambridge.

DoH (1992) *Local Voices.* Department of Health, London.

DoH (1997) *The New NHS.* Cm 3807. The Stationery Office, London.

Dolan JG (1995) Are patients capable of using the analytic hierarchy process and willing to use it to help make clinical decisions? *Medical Decision Making.* **15**(1): 76–80.

Dolan JG and Bordley DR (1993) Involving patients in complex decisions about their care – an approach using the analytic hierarchy process. *Journal of General Internal Medicine.* **8**(4): 204–9.

Dolan JG and Bordley DR (1994) Isoniazid prophylaxis – the importance of individual values. *Medical Decision Making.* **14**(1): 1–8.

Dolan P, Cookson R and Fergusson B (1999) Effect of discussion and deliberation on the public's views of priority setting in healthcare: focus group study. *British Medical Journal.* **318**: 916–19.

Dolan P, Gudex G, Kind P and Williams A (1995) The time trade-off method: results from a general population study. *Health Economics.* **5**(2): 141–54.

Doll RJ (1979) Consumers role in health-care costs. *Ohio State Medical Journal.* **75**(5): 301–3.

Donaldson C (1995) *Distributional aspects of willingness to pay.* Paper presented to the Health Economists Study Group, Aberdeen, July.

Donaldson C, Farrar S, Mapp T, Walker A and Macphee S (1997) Assessing community values in health care: is the willingness to pay method feasible? *Health Care Analysis.* **5**(1): 7–29.

Donovan J and Coast J (1994) Public preferences in priority-setting: unresolved issues. In: M Malek (ed) *Setting Priorities in Health Care.* John Wiley, Chichester.

Donovan J and Coast J (1996) Public participation in priority setting: commitment or illusion?. In J Coast, J Donovan and S Frankel (eds) *Priority Setting: The Health Care Debate.* John Wiley, Chichester.

Dougherty CJ (1991) *Setting health-care priorities: Oregon's next steps.* Hastings Center Report. **21**(3) suppl., pp 1–10.

Dowie J (1995) Personal communication.

Doyal L (1993) The role of the public in health care rationing. *Critical Public Health.* **4**(1): 49–54.

Doyal L (1995) How not to ration health care: the moral perils of utilitarian decision making. In: F Honigsbaum, J Richards and T Lockett (eds) *Priority Setting in Action.* Radcliffe Medical Press, Oxford.

Drummond MF, Stoddart GL and Torrance GW (1987) *Methods for the Economic Evaluation of Health Care Programmes.* Oxford Medical Publications, Oxford.

Duce R (1995) Court to decide on leukaemia girl's chance to live. *The Times,* 10 March.

Dumfries and Galloway Health Board (1992) *Needs Assessment 2: General Practitioners' Opinions of Health Services Available to Their Patients.* Department of Public Health Medicine, Dumfries.

Dumfries and Galloway Health Board (1994) *Needs Assessment 6: GP Survey 1994.* Department of Public Health Medicine, Dumfries.

Dunford A (1977) Planning for the consumer: the views of Community Health Councils. MA dissertation, Essex University.

Dunning AJ (1992) *Report of the Government Committee on Choices in Healthcare. Choices in Health Care.* Ministry of Welfare and Cultural Affairs, Rijswijk, The Netherlands.

Dyer RF and Forman EH (1992) Group decision support with the analytic hierarchy process. *Decision Support Systems.* **8**(2): 99–124.

Edgar W (1998) *Rationing health care in New Zealand – how the public have a say.* Paper presented to the Second International Conference on Priorities in Health Care, London.

Edwards J (1995) Public enemy: why asking the people about acute services goes wrong. *Health Services Journal.* **105**(5469): 22–4.

Edwards RT (1994) An economic perspective of the Salisbury waiting list points scheme. In: M Malek (ed) *Setting Priorities in Health Care.* John Wiley, Chichester.

Eltringham DM and Clare PH (1973) *Waiting List Management by Computer.* Operational Research Unit, Management Services Division, Birmingham Regional Hospital Board.

Elwyn GJ, Williams LA, Barry S and Kinnersley P (1996) Waiting list management in general practice: a review of orthopaedic patients. *British Medical Journal.* **312**: 887–8.

Emson HE (1991) Down the Oregon trail – the way for Canada? *Canadian Medical Association Journal.* **145**(11): 1441–3.

Enelow JM (1997) Cycling and majority rule. In: DC Mueller (ed) *Perspectives on Public Choice.* Cambridge University Press, Cambridge.

Entwistle VA, Sheldon TA, Sowden A and Watt IS (1998) Evidence-informed patient choice. *International Journal of Technology Assessment in Health Care.* **14**(2): 212–25.

Etzioni A (1991) Health-care rationing – a critical evaluation. *Health Affairs.* **10**(2): 88–95.

Evans JG (1991) Ageing and rationing: physiology not age should determine care. *British Medical Journal.* **303**: 869–70.

Evans JG (1993) Health care rationing and elderly people. In: M Tunbridge (ed) *Rationing of Health Care in Medicine*. Royal College of Physicians, London.

Evans JG (1997) Rationing health care by age – the case against. *British Medical Journal*. **314**(7083): 822–5.

Faulder C (1985) *Whose Body Is It? The Troubling Issue of Informed Consent*. Virago Press, London.

Feuerstein MT (1980) Community participation in evaluation: problems and potentials. *International Nursing Review*. **27**(6): 187–90.

Fleck LM (1992) Just health-care rationing – a democratic decision-making approach. *University of Pennsylvania Law Review*. **140**(5): 1597–636.

Fleck LM (1994a) Just caring: health reform and health care rationing. *Journal of Medicine and Philosophy*. **19**(5): 435–43.

Fleck LM (1994b) Just caring: Oregon, health care rationing, and informed democratic deliberation. *Journal of Medicine and Philosophy*. **19**(4): 367–88.

Fleck LM (1995a) Personal communication.

Fleck LM (1995b) Just caring: assisted suicide and health care rationing. *University of Detroit Mercy Law Review*. **72**(4): 873–99.

Fleck LM and Hogan AJ (1993) *Just Caring: Conflicting Rights, Uncertain Responsibilities – Report of the Interactive Computer Demonstration*. Center for Ethics and Humanities in the Life Sciences, Michigan State University.

Flynn R, Wilson G and Pickard S (1996) *Markets and Networks: Contracting in Community Health Services*. Open University Press, Buckingham.

Foreman A (1996) Health needs assessment. In: J Percy-Smith (ed) *Needs Assessment in Public Policy*. Open University Press, Buckingham.

Frankel S (1991) Health needs, health-care requirements, and the myth of infinite demand. *Lancet*. **337**(8757): 1588–90.

Frankfort-Nachmias C and Nachmias D (1996) *Research Methods in the Social Sciences*, 5th edn, Edward Arnold, London.

French S and Stewart T (1993) Manipulation of analyses. *Journal of Multi-criteria Decision Analysis*. **2**(2): 63.

Fries JF (1980) Aging, natural death, and the compression of morbidity. *New England Journal of Medicine*. **303**(3): 130–5.

Fries JF (1984) Aging, natural death, and the compression of morbidity. *New England Journal of Medicine*. **310**(10): 659–60.

Fries JF (1989) The compression of morbidity: near or far? *Milbank Quarterly*. **67**(2): 208–32.

Fries JF, Williams CA and Morfeld D (1992) Improvement in intergenerational health. *American Journal of Public Health*. **82**(1): 109–12.

Fuchs VR (1990) The health sector's share of the gross national product. *Science*. **247**(4942): 534–8.

Garland MJ (1992) Rationing in public: Oregon's priority-setting methodology. In: MA Strosberg *et al.* (eds) *Rationing America's Medical Care: The Oregon Plan and Beyond*. The Brookings Institution, Washington DC.

George V and Wilding P (1985) *Ideology and Social Welfare*. Routledge and Kegan Paul, London.

Gerard K and Mooney G (1993) QALY league tables: handle with care. *Health Economics*. **2**(1): 59–64.

Getzen TE (1992) Population aging and the growth of health expenditures. *Journal of Gerontology, Social Sciences*. **47**: S98–S101.

Goodman LA and Markowitz H (1952) Social welfare functions based on individual rankings. *American Journal of Sociology*. **58**: 257–62.

Gosfield AG (1976) Approaches of nine federal health agencies to patient rights and consumer participation. *Public Health Reports*. **91**: 403–5.

Greenberg RR and Nunamaker TR (1994) Integrating the analytic hierarchy process (AHP) into the multiobjective budgeting models of public sector organizations. *Socioeconomic Planning Sciences*. **28**(3): 197–206.

Grimshaw JM and Hutchinson A (1995) Clinical practice guidelines – do they enhance value for money? *British Medical Bulletin*. **51**(4): 927–40.

Gudex C, Williams A, Jourdan M *et al.* (1990) Prioritising waiting lists. *Health Trends*. **22**(3): 103–8.

Gwynedd CHCs (1994) *Public Consultation by the Gwynedd Community Health Councils in Response to Gwynedd Health Authority/Gwynedd Family Practitioner Services Authority Local Strategy for Health*. Gwynedd Community Health Councils, Llandudno, Caernarfon, Dolgellau and Llangefni.

Hackler C (1993) Health care reform in the United States. *Health Care Analysis*. **1**(1): 5–13.

Hadorn DC (1991a) The role of public values in setting health-care priorities. *Social Science and Medicine*. **32**(7): 773–81.

Hadorn DC (1991b) Setting health care priorities in Oregon. *Journal of the American Medical Association*. **265**(17): 2218–25.

Hadorn DC (1992) The problem of discrimination in health care priority setting. *Journal of the American Medical Association*. **268**(11): 1454–58.

Hadorn DC and Brook RH (1991) The health care resource allocation debate: defining our terms. *Journal of the American Medical Association*. **266**(23): 3328–31.

Hadorn DC and Holmes AC (1997) The New Zealand priority criteria project. Part 1: Overview. *British Medical Journal*. **314**(7074): 131–4.

Hall C (1997) Move to ration NHS fertility treatment. *Daily Telegraph*, 6 May.

Hall MA (1993) Informed consent to rationing decisions. *Milbank Quarterly*. **71**(4): 645–8.

Hall MA (1994) Disclosing rationing decisions: a reply to Paul S Appelbaum. *Milbank Quarterly*. **72**(2): 211–15.

Ham C (1993) Priority setting in the NHS: reports from six districts. *British Medical Journal*. **307**(6901): 435–8.

Ham C (1998) Resources and rationing in the NHS. In: Macpherson G (ed) *Our NHS: A Celebration of 50 Years*. BMJ Books, London.

Harris J (1985) *The Value of Life*. Routledge, London.

Harris J (1987) QALYfying the value of life. *Journal of Medical Ethics.* **13**(3): 117–23.

Harris J (1988) EQALYTY. In: P Byrne (ed) *Health, Rights and Resources: King's College Studies 1987–8*, King Edward's Hospital Fund for London.

Harrison A, Dixon J, New B and Judge K (1997) Can the NHS cope in future? *British Medical Journal.* **314**(7074): 139–42.

Harrison S (1997) Central government should have a greater role in rationing decisions: the case against. In: B New (ed) *Rationing – Talk and Action in Health Care.* King's Fund and BMJ Publishing Group, London.

Harrison S and Hunter DJ (1994) *Rationing Health Care.* Institute for Public Policy Research, London.

Hart JT (1994) *Feasible Socialism: The National Health Service, Past, Present and Future.* Socialist Health Association, London.

Hatch J (1978) The role of individuals and communities. Self-help and consumer participation in the development of health care systems. *Annals of the New York Academy of Science.* **310**: 49–56.

Hauser JR and Shugan SM (1980) Intensity measures of consumer preference. *Operations Research.* **28**: 278–320.

Havighurst CC (1992) Prospective self-denial – can consumers contract today to accept health-care rationing tomorrow? *University of Pennsylvania Law Review,* **140**(5): 1755–808.

Healthcare 2000 (1995) *UK Health and Healthcare Services.* Healthcare 2000, London.

Heginbotham C (1993) Healthcare priority setting: a survey of doctors, managers, and the general public. In: *Rationing in Action.* BMJ Publishing Group, London.

Heginbotham C (1997) Why rationing is inevitable in the NHS. In: New B (ed) *Rationing – Talk and Action in Health Care.* King's Fund and BMJ Publishing Group, London.

Heginbotham C and Ham C with Cochrane M and Richards J (1992) *Purchasing Dilemmas.* King's Fund College, London.

Heginbotham C, Atkinson S, Herbert E, Spiers H, Hunt P and Mouncer Y (1993) *History of Local Voices.* Research Paper No.9. NAHAT, Birmingham.

Hill M and Bramley G (1986) *Analysing Social Policy.* Blackwell, Oxford, Chapter 11.

Hogwood BW and Gunn LA (1984) *Policy Analysis in the Real World.* Oxford University Press, Oxford.

Hoinville G and Courtenay G (1979) Measuring consumer priorities. In: T O'Riordan and RC D'Arge (eds) *Progress in Resource Management and Environmental Planning.* Vol.1. John Wiley, Chichester.

Honigsbaum F (1991) *Who shall Live? Who shall Die? – Oregon's Health Financing Proposals.* King's Fund College Papers, King's Fund College, London.

Honigsbaum F, Richards J and Lockett T (1995) *Priority Setting in Action: Purchasing Dilemmas.* Radcliffe Medical Press, Oxford.

Hopton J and Dlugolecka M (1995) Patients' perceptions of need for primary health care services: useful for priority setting? *British Medical Journal.* **310**: 1237–40.

Huber GP (1974) Multi-attribute utility models: a review of field and field-like studies. *Management Science.* **20**(10): 1393–402.

Hunt P (1995) Counting the cost of the latest surgical strike. Letter to the Editor. *The Guardian,* 31 August.

Hunter D (1992) Careless talk costs lives. *Health Service Journal,* **102**(5301): 17.

Hunter D (1993a) *Rationing Dilemmas in Health Care.* Research Paper No.8. NAHAT, Birmingham.

Hunter DJ (1993b) Rationing and health gain. *Critical Public Health.* **4**(1): 27–33.

Hyland ME (1992) A reformulation of quality of life for medical science. *Quality of Life Research.* **1**: 267–72.

Hyland ME and Crocker G (1995) Validation of an asthma quality of life diary in a clinical trial. *Thorax.* **50**: 724–30.

Im M (1998) *Health priority-setting at district level.* PhD thesis, University of Birmingham.

Jecker NS (1991) Age-based rationing and women. *Journal of the American Medical Association.* **266**(21): 3012–15.

Jecker NS and Pearlman RA (1989) Ethical constraints on rationing medical-care by age. *Journal of the American Geriatrics Society.* **37**(11): 1067–75.

Jefferson TO and Demicheli V (1995) A panel priority rating exercise for the British Forces Germany health services market test. *Journal of the Royal Army Medical Corps.* **141**(1): 29–34.

Jennett B (1988) Medical ethics and economics in clinical decision making. In: G Mooney and A McGuire (eds) *Medical Ethics and Economics in Health Care.* Oxford University Press, Oxford.

Jensen RE (1986) Comparison of consensus methods for priority ranking problems. *Decision Sciences.* **17**(2): 195–211.

Johnson KN, Johnson RL, Edwards DK and Wheaton CA (1993) Public participation in wildlife management: opinions from public meetings and random surveys. *Wildlife Society Bulletin.* **21**(3): 218–25.

Johnson M (1974) Whose stranger am I? Or patients are really people. In: K Barnard and K Lee (eds) *NHS Reorganisation Issues and Prospects.* Nuffield Centre for Health Services Studies, University of Leeds.

Jonas S (1978) Limitation of community control of health facilities and services (editorial). *American Journal of Public Health.* **68**(6): 541–3.

Kaplan RM (1992) A quality-of-life approach to health resource allocation. In: MA Strosberg *et al.* (eds) *Rationing America's Medical Care: The Oregon Plan and Beyond.* The Brookings Institution, Oregon.

Kelly GA (1963) *A Theory of Personality: the Psychology of Personal Constructs.* Norton, New York.

Kelman HR (1976) Evaluation of health care quality by consumers. *International Journal of Health Services.* **6**(3): 431–41.

Kind P (1988) The development of health indices. In: G Teeling-Smith (ed) *Measuring Health: a Practical Approach.* John Wiley, Chichester.

Kitzhaber JA (1993) Rationing in action: prioritising health services in an era of limits: the Oregon experience. *British Medical Journal.* **307**(6900): 373–7.

Kitzhaber J and Kemmy AM (1995) On the Oregon trail. *British Medical Bulletin.* **51**(4): 808–18.

Kitzinger J (1996) Introducing focus groups. In: N Mays and C Pope (eds) *Qualitative Research in Health Care.* BMJ Publishing Group, London.

Klein R (1993) Dimensions of rationing: who should do what. *British Medical Journal.* **307**(3899): 309–11.

Klein R and Redmayne S (1992) *Patterns of Priorities – A Study of the Purchasing and Rationing Policies of Health Authorities.* Research Paper No. 7. NAHAT, Birmingham.

Klein R, Day P and Redmayne S (1995) Rationing in the NHS: the dance of the seven veils - in reverse. *British Medical Bulletin.* **51**(4): 769–80.

Knox PL (1977) Regional and local variations in priority preferences. *Urban Studies.* **14**: 103–7.

Koseki LK (1977) Consumer participation in health maintenance organisations. *Health and Social Work (Washington).* **2**(4): 51–69.

Lenaghan J (1996a) *Rationing and Rights in Health Care.* Institute for Public Policy Research, London.

Lenaghan J (1996b) Involving the public: report of a pilot citizens' jury. In: Lenaghan J (ed) *Rationing and Rights in Health Care.* Institute for Public Policy Research, London.

Lenaghan J (ed) (1997) *Hard Choices in Health Care. Healthcare Rights in Europe.* BMJ Publishing Group, London.

Lenaghan J, New B and Mitchell E (1997) Setting priorities: is there a role for citizens' juries? In: B New (ed) *Rationing: Talk and Action in Health Care.* BMJ Publishing Group and King's Fund, London.

Letwin O and Redwood J (1988) *Britain's Biggest Enterprise Ideas for Radical Reform of the NHS.* Centre for Policy Studies, London.

Light D (1995) Lecture given to graduate students at HSMC, University of Birmingham, 15 May.

Light D (1997) The real ethics of rationing. *British Medical Journal.* **315**(7100): 112–15.

Linstone HA and Turoff M (eds) (1975) *The Delphi Method: Techniques and Applications.* Addison-Wesley, New York.

Locker D and Dunt D (1978) Theoretical and methodological issues in sociological studies of consumer satisfaction with medical care. *Social Science and Medicine.* **12**: 285–92.

Lockwood M (1988) Quality of life and resource allocation. In: JM Bell and S Mendus (eds) *Philosophy and Medical Welfare.* Cambridge University Press, Cambridge.

Lomas J (1997) Reluctant rationers: public input to health care priorities. *Journal of Health Services Research Policy.* **2**(2): 1–8.

Luckman J, Mackenzie M and Stringer J (1969) *Management Policies for Large Ward Units.* Health Report No.1. Institute for Operational Research, London.

Lupton C, Peckham S and Taylor P (1988) *Managing Public Involvement in Healthcare Purchasing*. Open University Press, Buckinghamshire.

Lutton GL (1992) *Choices in health care: a survey of lay and professional views*. Masters dissertation, Middlesex University.

MacDonald LD (1994) *Acute Services Community Survey*. Report to East Surrey Health Authority. Department of Public Health Services, St George's Hospital Medical School.

MacKay K (1996) Rationing health care. *British Medical Journal*. **313**(7056): 557.

Maynard A (1996a) Lean, mean rationing machine. *Health Service Journal*. **106**(5488): 21.

Maynard A (1996b) Rationing health care. *British Medical Journal*. **313**(7071): 1499.

McGee HM, O'Boyle CA, Hickey A, O'Malley K and Joyce CRB (1991) Assessing the quality of life of the individual: the SEIQoL with a healthy and a gastroenterology unit population. *Psychological Medicine*. **21**: 749–59.

McIver S (1997) Involving the public as citizens. *Health Services Management Centre Newsletter*. **3**(1): 1–2.

McIver S (1998) *Healthy Debate: an Independent Evaluation of Citizens' Juries*. King's Fund, London.

McLean I (1987) *Public Choice*. Blackwell, Oxford.

Mechanic D (1985) Cost containment and the quality of medical care: rationing strategies in an era of constrained resources. *Milbank Memorial Fund Quarterly*. **63**(3): 453–75.

Meddin J, Coventry A, Boldy D and Liveris M (1990) Evaluating consumer and provider participation in health-services policy, planning, and management – a Western Australian case-study. *Evaluation Review*. **14**(2): 134–50.

Menzel PT (1990) *Strong Medicine*. Oxford University Press, New York.

Menzel PT (1992) Oregon's denial: disabilities and quality of life. *Hastings Center Report*. **22**(6): 21–5.

Millet I (1997) The effectiveness of alternative preference elucidation methods in the analytic hierarchy process. *Journal of Multi-criteria Decision Analysis*. **6**(1): 41–51.

Milman A (1993) Maximizing the value of focus group research: qualitative analysis of consumers' destination choice. *Journal of Travel Research*. **32**(2): 61–4.

Mishra R (1984) *Society and Social Policy*. 2nd edn. Macmillan, Basingstoke.

Modolo M-A and Figa-Talamanca I (1977) Interaction between consumers and providers in health services: new roles and their implications. *International Journal of Health Education*. **20**(1): 41–4.

Mooney G (1989) QALYs: are they enough? A health economist's perspective. *Journal of Medical Ethics*. **15**: 148–52.

Mooney G, Gerard K, Donaldson C and Farrar S (1992) *Priority Setting in Purchasing*. Research Paper No. 6, NAHAT, Birmingham.

Mooney G, Jan S and Wiseman V (1995) Examining preferences for allocating health care gains. *Health Care Analysis*. **3**(3): 261–5.

Moore W (1996) *Hard Choices: Priority Setting in the NHS*. NAHAT, Birmingham.

Mueller DC (1997) Public choice in perspective. In: DC Mueller (ed) *Perspectives on Public Choice*. Cambridge University Press, Cambridge.

Mullen PM (1983) *Delphi-type Studies in the Health Services: the Impact of the Scoring System*. Health Services Management Centre, Research Report 17, University of Birmingham.

Mullen PM (1994) Waiting lists in the post-review NHS. *Health Services Management Research*. **7**(2): 131–45.

Mullen PM, Murray-Sykes K and Kearns WE (1982) *CHC Involvement in District Planning Teams: Policy and Politics and Practice*. HSMC Research Report 15, University of Birmingham.

Mullen PM, Murray-Sykes K and Kearns WE (1984) Community Health Council representation on planning teams: a question of politics. *Public Health*. **98**(2): 143–51.

Mullin J (1995) Father sees hope for leukaemia girl vanish in volte-face. *The Guardian*, 11 March.

Murray AF and Berrill A (1975) Improving citizen feedback. *Nations Cities Journal*. 36–8.

Murray SA, Tapson J, Turnbull L, McCallum J and Little A (1994) Listening to local voices: adapting rapid appraisal to assess health and social needs in general practice. *British Medical Journal*. **308**: 698–700.

National Advisory Committee on Core Health and Disability Support Services (1992) *Best of Health*. Ministry of Health, Wellington, New Zealand.

Nelson RM and Drought T (1992) Justice and the moral acceptability of rationing medical care – the Oregon experiment. *Journal of Medicine and Philosophy*. **17**(1): 97–117.

New B (on behalf of the Rationing Agenda Group) (1996) The rationing agenda in the NHS. *British Medical Journal*. **312**: 1593–601.

New B (1997) Defining a package of healthcare services the NHS is responsible for – the case for. *British Medical Journal*. **314**: 503–5.

New B and Le Grand J (1996) *Rationing in the NHS: Principles and Pragmatism*. King's Fund, London.

NHSE (1996a) *Priorities and Planning Guidance 1997/98*. NHS Executive, Leeds.

NHSE (1996b) *Patient Partnership: Building a Collaborative Strategy*. NHSE, London.

NHSE, Institute of Health Services Management and NHS Confederation (1998) *In the Public Interest: Developing a Strategy for Public Participation in the NHS*. Bridge Consultancy, Cambridge.

Nord E (1990) A comment on the meaning of numerical valuations of health states. *Social Science and Medicine*. **30**(8): 943–4.

Nord E (1993) Unjustified use of the Quality of Well-Being Scale in priority setting in Oregon. *Health Policy*. **24**(1): 45–53.

Norheim OF (1995) The Norwegian welfare state in transition: rationing and plurality of values as ethical challenges for the health care system. *Journal of Medicine and Philosophy*. **20**(6): 639–55.

O'Brien B and Viramontes JL (1994) Willingness to pay: a valid and reliable measure of health state preference? *Medical Decision Making.* **14**(3): 288–97.

Observer (1995) Twinned questions of life and death. Editorial. *The Observer,* 17 September.

OECD (1993) *OECD Health Systems: Facts and Trends 1960–1991, Volume 1.* OECD, Paris.

Ong BN and Humphris G (1994) Prioritizing needs with communities: rapid appraisal methodologies in health. In: J Popay and G Williams (eds) *Researching the People's Health.* Routledge, London.

Ong BN, Humphris G, Annett H and Rifkin S (1991) Rapid appraisal in an urban setting, an example from the developed world. *Social Science and Medicine.* **32**(8): 909–15.

Paap WR (1978) Consumer-based boards of health centres: structural problems in achieving effective control. *American Journal of Public Health.* **68**(6): 578–82.

Paap WR and Hanson B (1979) Comment on Jonas editorial on consumer involvement. *American Journal of Public Health.* **69**(2): 179.

Parahoo K (1997) *Nursing Research: Principles, Process and Practice.* Macmillan, Basingstoke.

Parker RA (1967) Social administration and scarcity: the problem of rationing. *Social Work.* **24**(2): 9–14.

Pateman C (1970) *Participation and Democratic Theory.* Cambridge University Press, Cambridge.

Pattanaik PK (1997) Some paradoxes of preference aggregation. In: DC Mueller (ed) *Perspectives on Public Choice.* Cambridge University Press, Cambridge.

Pawlson LG, Glover JJ and Murphy DJ (1992) An overview of allocation and rationing – implications for geriatrics. *Journal of the American Geriatrics Society.* **40**(6): 628–34.

Perez J (1994) Theoretical elements of comparison among ordinal discrete multicriteria methods. *Journal of Multi-criteria Decision Analysis.* **3**(3): 157–76.

Perez J and Barbra-Romero S (1995) Three practical criteria of comparison among ordinal preference aggregating rules. *European Journal of Operational Research.* **85**(3): 473–87.

Phoenix CJ (1972) Waiting list management and admission scheduling. In: ME Abrams (ed) *Spectrum 71: A Conference on Medical Computing.* Butterworths, London.

Pollitt C (1986) Beyond the managerial model: the case for broadening performance assessment in government and the public services. *Financial Accountability and Management.* **2**(3): 155–70.

Pollock A (1992) Local voices: the bankruptcy of the democratic process. *British Medical Journal.* **305**(6853): 535–6.

Pollock AM (1995) Review of 'Priority Setting Processes for Health Care': Honigsbaum *et al. British Medical Journal.* **310**(6877): 474–5.

Posnett J (1993) The political economy of health care reform in the UK. In: RJ Arnould,

RF Rich and WN White (eds) *Competitive Approaches to Health Care Reform*. The Urban Institute Press, Washington DC.

Price D (1996) Lessons for health care rationing from the case of child B. *British Medical Journal*. **312**(7024): 167–9.

Rabinowitz J (1992) Collective decision-making: the analytic hierarchy process. *Social Policy and Administration*. **36**(1): 87–97.

Rae DW and Schickler E (1997) Majority rule. In: DC Mueller (ed) *Perspectives on Public Choice*. Cambridge University Press, Cambridge.

Rawles J (1989) Castigating QALYs. *Journal of Medical Ethics*. **15**: 143–7.

RCP (1995) *Setting Priorities in the NHS*. Royal College of Physicians, London.

Reagan MD (1990) Health care rationing and cost containment are not synonymous. *Policy Studies Review*. **9**(2): 219–23.

Redmayne S (1992) Skin deep. *Health Service Journal*. **102**(5325): 28–9.

Redmayne S and Klein R (1993) Rationing in practice: the case of in vitro fertilisation. *British Medical Journal*. **306**(6891): 1521–4.

Relman A (1990) Is rationing inevitable? *New England Journal of Medicine*. **322**: 1809–10.

Richardson A (1983) *Participation*. Routledge and Kegan Paul, London.

Richardson A, Charny M and Hammer-Lloyd S (1992) Public opinion and purchasing. *British Medical Journal*. **304**(6828): 680–2.

Rivlin MM (1997) Can age-based rationing of health care be morally justified? *Mount Sinai Journal of Medicine*. **64**(2): 113–19.

Roberts C, Crosby D, Dunn R *et al.* (1995a) Blind to the nature of life itself. *Health Service Journal*. **105**(5454): 21.

Roberts C, Crosby D, Dunn R *et al.* (1995b) Rational rather than rationed. *Health Service Journal*. **105**(5464): 17.

Roberts C, Crosby D, Grundy P *et al.* (1996) The wasted millions. *Health Service Journal*. **106**(5524): 24–7.

Robinson R (1997) Rationing health care: a national framework and local discretion. *Journal of Health Services Research and Policy*. **2**(2): 67–70.

Rothermel MA and Schilling DA (1984) A comparative study of three methods of eliciting preference information. *OMEGA*. **12**(4): 379–89.

Rutt HM (1997) *The public interest in decision-making*. PhD thesis, University of Birmingham.

Ryan M (1996a) Using willingness to pay to assess the benefits of assisted reproductive techniques. *Health Economics*. **5**(6): 543–58.

Ryan M (1996b) *Using Consumer Preferences in Health Care Decision Making: the Application of Conjoint Analysis*. Office of Health Economics, London.

Ryan M and Hughes J (1997) Using conjoint analysis to assess women's preference for miscarriage management. *Health Economics*. **6**(3): 261–73.

Saaty TL (1977) A scaling method for priorities in hierarchical structures. *Journal of Mathematical Psychology*. **15**(3): 234–81.

Saaty TL (1997) That is not the analytic hierarchy process: what the AHP is and what it is not. *Journal of Multi-Criteria Decision Analysis.* **6**(6): 324–35.

Saaty TL and Alexander JM (1980) *Thinking with Models.* Pergamon Press, Oxford.

Sackett D (1996) *The Doctor's (Ethical and Economic) Dilemma.* Office of Health Economics, London.

Salter B (1993) The politics of purchasing in the National Health Service. *Policy and Politics.* **21**(3): 171–84.

Salter B (1994) Change in the British National Health Service: policy paradox and the rationing issue. *International Journal of Health Services.* **24**(1): 45–72.

Sancar FH (1993) An integrative approach to public participation and knowledge generation in design. *Landscape and Urban Planning.* **26**(1/4): 67–88.

Scheerder R (1993) Dutch choices in health care. In: *Rationing in Action.* BMJ Publishing Group, London.

Schneider EL and Brody JA (1983) Aging, natural death, and the compression of morbidity. *New England Journal of Medicine.* **309**(14): 854–6.

Shackley P and Ryan M (1995) Involving consumers in health care decision making. *Health Care Analysis.* **3**(3): 196–204.

Singleton P (1994) *Healthy Havering Project.* Public Health Research Report No.23. Directorate of Public Health Medicine, Barking and Havering Health Authority.

SMSR (1994) *Summary of Public Consultation Days undertaken by Derbyshire Family Health Services Authority, Southern Derbyshire Health Authority and Derbyshire Social Services.* Social and Market Survey Research Ltd, Hull.

Spurgeon P (1993) Regulation or free market for the NHS? A case for co-existence. In: I Tilly (ed) *Managing The Internal Market.* Paul Chapman Publishing, London.

Spurgeon P (1997) The experience of contracting in healthcare. In: R Flynn and G Williams (eds) *Contracting for Health: Quasi Markers and the National Health Service.* Oxford University Press, Oxford.

Spurgeon P (1998) *Values and attitudes affecting public involvement.* Paper presented to the Second International Conference on Priorities in Health Care, London.

Stewart J (1995) *Innovation in Democratic Practice.* INLOGOV, University of Birmingham.

Stewart J, Kendall E and Coote A (1994) *Citizens' Juries.* Institute for Public Policy Research, London.

Stimson DH (1971) Health agency decision making: an operations research perspective. In: MF Arnold, LV Blankenship and J Hess (eds) *Administrative Health Systems: Issues and Perspectives.* Aldine Atherton, Chicago and New York.

Strauss RP and Hughes GD (1976) A new approach to the demand for public goods. *Journal of Public Economics.* **6**: 191–204.

Swedish Parliamentary Priorities Commission (1995) *Priorities in Health Care.* Swedish Government Official Reports 1995:5. The Ministry of Health and Social Affairs, Stockholm.

Tideman TN (1997) Voting and the revelation of preferences for public activities. In: DC Mueller (ed) *Perspectives on Public Choice.* Cambridge University Press, Cambridge.

Torrance GW (1986) Measurement for health state utilities for economic appraisal. *Journal of Health Economics*. **5**(1): 1–30.

Torrance GW and Feeney D (1989) Utilities and quality-adjusted life years. *International Journal of Technology Assessment in Health Care*. **5**: 559–75.

Toth B (1996) Public participation: an historical perspective. In: J Coast, J Donovan and S Frankel (eds) *Priority Setting: the Health Care Debate*. John Wiley, Chichester.

Triantaphyllou E, Lootsma FA, Pardalos PM and Mann SH (1994) On the evaluation and application of different scales for quantifying pairwise comparisons in fuzzy sets. *Journal of Multi-criteria Decision Analysis*. **3**(3): 133–55.

Turksen IB and Willson IA (1994) A fuzzy set preference model for consumer choice. *Fuzzy Sets and Systems*. **68**(3): 253–66.

Turley J (1995) The inhuman rationing of health care. Letter to the Editor. *The Guardian*, 14 March.

Van den Heuval WJ (1980) The role of the consumer in health policy. *Social Science and Medicine*. **14A**(5): 423–5.

Van de Ven WPMM (1995) Choices in health care: a contribution from The Netherlands. *British Medical Bulletin*. **51**(4): 781–90.

Veatch RM (1992) The Oregon experience: needless and real worries. In: MA Strosberg *et al*. (eds) *Rationing America's Medical Care: The Oregon Plan and Beyond*. The Brookings Institution, Washington DC.

Victor P and Penman D (1995) New NHS-speak has no word for compassion. *Independent on Sunday*, 12 March.

Victor P, Penman D and Castle S (1995) Anonymous donor pays for Girl B's treatment. *Independent on Sunday*, 12 March.

Walley T and Barton S (1995) A purchaser perspective of managing new drugs: interferon beta as a case study. *British Medical Journal*. **311**: 796–9.

Ward D (1993) Smoker dies after operation was denied until he gave up. *The Guardian*, 17 August.

Weale A (1979) Statistical lives and the principle of maximum benefit. *Journal of Medical Ethics*. **5**: 185–95.

Weale A (1990) The allocation of scarce medical resources: a democrat's dilemma. In: P Byrne (ed) *Medicine, Medical Ethics and the Value of Life*. John Wiley, Chichester.

Weale A (1995a) The ethics of rationing. *British Medical Bulletin*. **51**(4): 831–41.

Weale A (1998) Rationing health care. *British Medical Journal*. **316**(7129): 410.

Weale S (1995b) Dying girl refused NHS treatment. *The Guardian*, 10 March.

Welch HG and Larson EB (1988) Dealing with limited resources: the Oregon decision to curtail funding for organ transplantation. *New England Journal of Medicine*. **319**: 171–3.

Whitty P (1992) *What are Colchester People's Priorities for Health Care? A Population Survey in Urban Colchester*. North Essex Health Authority.

Wiener JM (1992) Rationing in America: overt and covert. In: MA Strosberg *et al*. (eds) *Rationing America's Medical Care: The Oregon Plan and Beyond*. The Brookings Institution, Washington DC.

Williams A (1988) *Priority Setting in Public and Private Health Care: A Guide through the Ideological Jungle.* Discussion Paper 36. Centre for Health Economics, University of York.

Williams A (1995) Economics, QALYs and medical ethics – a health economist's perspective. *Health Care Analysis.* **3**(3): 221–6.

Williams A (1997) Intergenerational equity: an exploration of the fair innings argument. *Health Economics.* **6**(2): 117–32.

Williams MH and Frankel SJ (1993) The myth of infinite demand. *Critical Public Health.* **4**(1): 13–18.

Wilson G (1991) Models of ageing and their relation to policy formation and service provision. *Policy and Politics.* **19**(1): 37–47.

Wordsworth S, Donaldson C and Scott A (1996) *Can We Afford the NHS?* Institute of Public Policy Research, London.

Zimmern R (1995) *Challenging Choices.* 2nd Annual Report of the Director of Health Policy and Public Health for Cambridge and Huntingdon Health Commission.

Index

Milton Keynes UK
Ingram Content Group UK Ltd.
UKHW051926141024
449569UK00027B/1372